Freedom with Food and Fitness

Alana Van Der Sluys

Freedom with Food and Fitness

How Intuitive Eating is the Key to Your Happiest, Healthiest Self.

Urano
publishing

Argentina - Chile - Colombia - Spain
USA - Mexico - Peru - Uruguay

Urano
publishing

Cover art and design by Luis Tinoco

Cover copyright © Urano Publishing, an imprint of Urano World USA, Inc

The first edition of this book was published in November 2023

ISBN: 978-1-953027-19-1

E-ISBN: 978-1-953027-20-7

Printed in Spain

Library of Cataloging-in-Publication Data

Van Der Sluys, Alana

1. Health & Wellness   2. Diet & Exercise

Freedom with Food and Fitness

Dedication

To Archer: I love you the whole sun, stars, moon, and universe.

Acknowledgements

"One is too small a number to achieve greatness. No accomplishment of real value has ever been achieved by a human being working alone."

–JOHN C. MAXWELL

There are countless people and interactions that shape who we become. I would be remiss not to acknowledge and show my deepest gratitude to those who helped me become someone who could write her truth in a public way and find the means to show it to the world. I am forever grateful to those who made the conscious decision to support me in achieving one of my biggest dreams. I hope this book will be the first of many so I can continue to speak my truth; share my passions; and help those who struggle with food, weight, and self-worth all around the world.

First, to my parents, Jo-Ann and William Rome, who raised me to believe that my best is always enough, that being a woman is not a hindrance, and that everyone is worthy of love and respect. You never once dissuaded me from pursuing my passions nor questioned my capabilities. Thank you, and I love you.

To my husband, Scott, who took loving me "in sickness and in health" to heart, even though we didn't write it in our wedding vows. You've never judged me at my worst, and you've always been willing to weather the storm with me, as I have for you. Thank you for being my best friend. I love you.

To my son, Archer: One of my biggest motivations to heal my relationship with myself was to be able to teach you how not to strain your relationship with yourself. I wanted to show you what a self-assured woman looks like and how she shows up with authenticity and self-compassion. I want you, who will be socialized as a man, to see yourself as worthy, too, no matter what you accomplish. You are, unequivocally, the most important thing in my life. I will love, support, and hold space for you unconditionally, forever.

To my developmental editor, Lydia Stevens, and my literary agent, Elaine Spencer, at The Knight Agency: thank you for taking a chance on a small fish in a very big pond.

To all those who donated to my book fund back when I thought I would have to publish the book on my own: my aunts and uncles Gina and Rich Perrone, Linda and Rafik Cezanne, and Karen and Joe Tesoriero; my cousins Kim and April Tesoriero; friends Samantha Lake, Richard DiMaio, Christina Newton, my "big brother" Mike and his wife Carol Augustyni, Diana and Bobby Smillie, Brenda Adames, and Elizabeth O'Connor.

To my mentors: Evelyn Tribole, Elyse Resch, Christy Harrison, Maria Scrimenti, Jenna Free, Lauren Mcaulay, Caroline Dooner, Rachel Hollis, Brooke Castillo, and Jessi Jean. Thank you for giving me the knowledge and strength to heal myself and the inspiration to help heal others. I have yet to meet any of you in person, but that only speaks to the power of the work you do.

And finally, to all my other family, friends, clients, and followers on social media: you know who you are, and I hope you know how much I love and appreciate you.

Table of Contents

Introduction

There are many who think "seeing is believing." I've heard this adage frequently, mostly when people talk of UFOs, ghosts, and religion. I used to believe it, too. If something was in front of my eyes, it must be real; it must be true.

Then came Photoshop. And Instagram filters. All of a sudden, I couldn't trust what I saw with my own two eyes because what was in front of me was no longer real.

Unfortunately, our brains are designed to interpret whatever we see in front of us as such. We see "perfect" bodies—tapered waists, glistening muscles, smooth unblemished skin—and we take these images at face value, pun intended. We compare ourselves to them, these impossible standards, and adopt disordered behaviors in the futile attempt to achieve these aesthetic goals. I know this because I've lived it; and if you're reading these words, chances are you have, too.

The Philosophy Behind *Freedom with Food and Fitness* and the Ten Principles of Intuitive Eating

I found recovery from my disordered eating through a philosophy called intuitive eating. Although the concept is incredibly nuanced, intuitive eating is, simply put, listening to and honoring your body's unique needs, cravings, and energy levels with regard to food and movement. This anti-diet philosophy not only stands on the foundation of ten core principles, but is also an "evidence-based model with a validated assessment scale and over 100 studies to date," according to its founders, registered dietitian Evelyn Tribole and nutrition therapist Elyse Resch. In order to truly get the most out of this book and its tried-and-true, by yours truly, strategies for food and body peace, you first need to know those ten principles.

1. *Reject the Diet Mentality* – Quiet the noise of media and society that says you need to be thin, fit, muscular, or otherwise "perfect." Social media has made these messages even more pervasive, and as a result, more difficult to filter from our personal narratives. This principle suggests that you do a media detox; weed out as many harmful and disordered messages as you can and replace them with ones that promote true health, happiness, and acceptance. These types of accounts center on intuitive eating, health at every size, weight neutrality, body neutrality, body liberation and anti-diet; and do a "gut check." If you follow a social media account or read a magazine and it makes you feel as if you are less than or a problem that needs to be fixed, ditch it. Unfollow or light it on fire, respectively.

2. *Honor Your Hunger* – Eat when you're hungry—and there are many different kinds of hunger! Hunger is a biological cue that your body needs energy and nourishment. Many timed nutrition or intermittent fasting diets promote arbitrary "ideal" times to eat, but what happens when you're hungry *now*? Do you wait two hours until your designated eating time, increasingly fixated on how hungry you are and the food you want to eat? Or do you just honor your hunger and eat? You guessed it—you just eat. Ignoring your hunger signals typically leads to

a sharp drop in blood sugar. This drop in blood sugar can mess with your ability to choose foods that will nourish your body in two ways: first, low blood sugar leads to brain fog, so the ability to make sound decisions is impaired; and second, your brain will tell you to choose a food high in sugar or carbs in order to bring your blood sugar back up. While there is nothing inherently wrong with foods that have sugar or carbs, by themselves they will do little to nourish or satisfy you until your next meal.

3. *Make Peace with Food* – Give yourself unconditional permission to eat. You can eat whatever you want, whenever you want, in what-ever quantity you want. You are an autonomous adult. The reason you are afraid you would eat a whole tub of ice cream if you gave yourself unconditional permission is because you've been denying yourself ice cream for so long! Exposing yourself to foods you fear or find triggering, known as habituation, will, ironically, decrease the urge to binge on them. It's like when your partner says, "I love you" for the first time. You get butterflies! Ten years down the road, it's still lovely to hear, but it doesn't elicit the same intense emotion. The same can be applied to trigger foods through frequent and un-conditional exposure.

For those who are emotional overeaters, habituation may only be one piece of the puzzle. In this case, it can be explored simultaneously with cognitive behavioral therapy (CBT). CBT can include a variety of modalities, including role playing, journaling, thought reframing, and relaxation techniques. These are methods I use with my clients, as much of the work of recovery is mindset work and emotional management.

4. *Challenge the Food Police* – The Food Police is the version of diet culture that lives in your head. It's the one insisting that certain foods

or behaviors around food are "good" or "bad," "healthy" or "unhealthy." In addition to the outside voices that you need to quiet, your inner critic needs to be told to pipe down, too.

5. *Discover the Satisfaction Factor* – Food can be pleasurable, as can the entire experience of going out to eat with family and friends! These experiences can be stripped of their enjoyment when diet culture makes you afraid of food and your body's natural cues. You *can* enjoy delicious food without guilt and you *can* become in tune with your satisfaction in terms of what you eat and how much. If I eat a whole bag of frozen cauliflower, I might become physically full, but I certainly won't be satiated because I would not find pleasure in the experience. On the other hand, I can have one or two cookies and feel completely satiated, without any guilt.

6. *Feel Your Fullness* – Many disordered eaters experience binge-restrict cycles: they restrict calories in the name of a diet or weight loss, only to experience a binge on the very foods they were denying themselves. This leads not only to emotional feelings of guilt and shame, but also to physical feelings of bloating or uncomfortable fullness. This can be a vicious cycle, particularly for those who cope with negative emotions through eating. If the binge leads to shame, feelings of shame can then lead to more bingeing, and on and on. With intuitive eating, though, you effortlessly stop eating when you're physically full and satiated.

7. *Cope with Your Emotions with Kindness* – With this principle, you learn that negative emotions can be valuable learning tools, so you do not bury them or push them away. You can use a variety of "thought work" tools to manage how you feel around food, your body, and your weight. There are so many emotions that crop up during this

journey to freedom and recovery, both positive and negative, you need tools to know how to manage and utilize them.

8. *Respect Your Body* – Dieting will get you a different body. That is almost certain. But for how long? And at what cost? There are also the factors of genetics, metabolic rate, and nutritional needs in determining one's unique body size and shape. With this principle, you learn to respect your body as it is, instead of manipulating or punishing it when it's not as malleable as you hoped it would be, or as diet culture told you it could be.

9. *Movement—Feel the Difference* – Movement, exercise, fitness: whatever you call it, the incorporation of physical activity is what differentiates *Freedom with Food and Fitness* from other books on intuitive eating. Physical activity *does* have a place in recovery, so long as it doesn't become a trigger and is not the focal point of your disorder. For some going through recovery, they may see physical activity as a way either to "earn" food they want to eat but feel they shouldn't, or to make up for food they've already eaten, for which they feel guilt. When fitness is used to balance the scales of eating, literally and figuratively, or for the sole purpose of manipulating the body's shape or making it smaller, it can become a hindrance to recovery. The second half of this book explores different types of movement, what type is best for you, and, if you want them, how to set fitness goals that, like your relationship with food, come from a place of self-love and not punishment.

10. *Honor Your Health With Gentle Nutrition* – Many scoff at intuitive eating, believing it is a philosophy that allows people to give up on their health or promotes obesity. Typically "obesity" is seen as an offensive term, but I use it here to mimic the language of skeptics; these

people tend to forget, or never even know about, this final, and crucial, principle. As an intuitive eater, you will honor cravings and eat delicious, satisfying meals, but you will also consider how you will feel after the meal. You will be in tune with your body *before, during, and after* you eat and choose foods you know will leave you feeling energized and satiated.

This book is divided into two parts: food and fitness. While I wholeheartedly believe in the philosophy of intuitive eating and its principles, I also believe that philosophies and principles, as abstract concepts, aren't enough to face your diet demons. You need explicit, actionable strategies and tips that you can implement as soon as today.

What also sets *Freedom with Food and Fitness* apart from other intuitive eating books is that I teach you how to reclaim the tools hijacked by diet culture for your own food freedom. For example, you don't need to abandon meal prepping, especially if you work long hours outside of the home, but you don't need to stick to rigid schedules as a way to control your eating. We can use general knowledge of macronutrients to build nourishing and satisfying meals, instead of weighing our food and counting our grams.

Nothing is inherently healthy or unhealthy. What makes something healthy or unhealthy has everything to do with intention and mindset, which is what we will explore here.

My Journey from Disorder to Freedom

Trigger warning: I use calorie numbers to discuss my journey from eating disorder to recovery.

Although I'll delve with greater detail into how perfectionism and its manifestation of disordered eating had, ironically, made my life way less than perfect, I'll start with a general synopsis of how I got here, writing this book for you, and, let's be honest, a little for me.

I grew up as the only child in my household. Both my parents came from modest upbringings and made it their life's mission to give me what they never had by providing me with every opportunity I could ever ask for. As a result, I was praised a lot as a child; and no, it wasn't "everyone's a winner." Although given ample opportunities and praise, I worked hard for what I wanted. I also failed a lot and was allowed the opportunity to do so.

It was easy to be praised as a big fish in a small pond, otherwise known as rural upstate New York. I was conventionally pretty—long brown hair, thin frame, big brown eyes—and I excelled in most school subjects and extracurricular activities. I became accustomed to being praised and externally validated for being "the good girl," rule follow-ing, and people pleasing. Over time, I developed what Brene Brown, defines as perfectionism: "a self-destructive and addictive belief system that fuels this primary thought: If I look perfect and do everything perfectly, I can avoid or minimize the painful feelings of blame, judg-ment, and shame."

My life until college was more or less on the same trajectory. Life came easy. Although I worked diligently for my accomplishments, I didn't have any roadblocks either. Call it white privilege. Call it thin privilege. Call it middle class privilege. Call it whatever you want. There will be more on that privilege in terms of writing this book in a bit.

By the time I got to graduate school, I had abandoned my first dream of becoming a journalist after receiving a bachelor's degree in journal-ism; it turned out being a rookie music journalist would likely result in living paycheck to paycheck with an unsteady work schedule. For some-one who craved stability and predictability, because it had worked so well for me up until that point, the idea of a seemingly unstable career path made my skin itch. My teenage brain and underdeveloped prefrontal cortex figured, at the time, that a love of rock music and writing would be enough to recreate the lifestyle I was accustomed to, in adulthood.

I stayed in college to earn a master's degree, this time in English education. As I was finishing up this second degree, I realized that, for the first time in my life, I didn't know what my future held. It was easy when I knew I had the grades, the friends, and the identity of "student." Now, I was being thrust into the workforce: no idea where I would teach or whether I would even land a job in time for September, where I would live, and if I'd be separated from everyone I'd known. For someone who always had control over her life, this was terrifying. My life's compass had guided me expertly until this point, and now it felt as if it was in a perpetual state of rerouting.

I know what you're thinking: not-so-poor little entitled girl who never had to deal with real issues like poverty, prejudice, broken homes, abuse ... and you're right. I'll be the first to admit that, relatively speaking, I've led a privileged life, and the problem of not being in control of where my life was heading next, armed with my expensive degrees and supportive parents, no less, would be most other people's idea of winning the lottery.

But we approach life through our own lived experience, and that was my experience. To me, it was terrifying. Despite different life circumstances, we've *all* felt scared and lost in one way or another; it's the human condition. We've all felt out of control and at the mercy of fate or others around us. We've all felt like we're drowning, that time is moving forward, and there's not a thing we can do to stop it. We've all been scared to make a mistake, to misstep. We, as humans, share this fear of powerlessness, that our lives are not ours to navigate.

I craved control of something. Anything.

And like most young girls and women—and yes, even some men—today do, I took control of my weight.

I developed an eating disorder.

Contrary to what most people believe, those with eating disorders don't always fit the stereotypical waif-thin white girl, with slouching posture, stringy hair hanging over her bony shoulders, skin taut against sunken cheekbones, brittle nails attached to white knuckles that are resisting the blinding urge to reach for the most minute amount of food. Eating disorders affect all races, genders, sexual orientations, religions, social standings, and body types. According to a meta-analysis of 36 studies, only six percent of people with eating disorders are medically diagnosed as "underweight," which means most people with eating disorders are either at normal weight, overweight, or obese, according to Body Mass Index (BMI) standards. [1] What's more, black teenagers are fifty percent more likely than white teenagers to exhibit bulimic behavior, such as binge eating and purging. [2] Gay men are seven times more likely to report binge eating and twelve times more likely to report purging than heterosexual men. While the data on how eating disorders affect people of all types is much more vast than three studies, clearly the problem spans far wider than popular media would suggest.

As I'm sharing my experience with you, it feels like the right time to discuss the difference between an eating disorder and disordered eating. An eating disorder is typically a condition formally diagnosed by a mental health professional and falls in line with the criteria found in the DSM-5 (*The Diagnostic and Statistical Manual of Mental Disorders*,

---

1. Jon Arcelus, Alex J. Mitchell, Jackie Wales, et al., "Mortality Rates in Patients with Anorexia Nervosa and Other Eating Disorders: A Meta-analysis of 36 Studies," *Archives of General Psychiatry* 68, no. 7 (2011): 724–31.

2. Anne E. Becker, Debra L. Franko, Alexandra Speck, and David B. Herzog, "Ethnicity and Differential Access to Care for Eating Disorder Symptoms," *International Journal of Eating Disorders* 33, no. 2 (March 2003): 205–12.

Fifth Edition). I suffered from binge eating disorder (BED), which results in binge—restrict cycles and intense feelings of guilt and shame. Fueling my BED was body dysmorphic disorder (BDD), where one fixates on the perceived flaws of a particular body part; in my case, my abdominal area.

On the other hand, disordered eaters exhibit similar behaviors to those with eating disorders but with less severity. Disordered eating can include behaviors like obsessively weighing yourself, measuring food, macros and calorie counting, yo-yo dieting, weight cycling, and preoccupation with thoughts of food. The line between disordered eating and an eating disorder is thin; the slope is slippery. Do not let anyone, including yourself, tell you that you're not sick enough to seek help if you feel you need it. Everyone's experience is valid.

In addition to BED, I suffered from orthorexia, an obsession with eating only "healthy, clean" food; at the time of this writing, orthorexia is not included in the DSM-5, but it is widely recognized by mental health professionals as a form of disordered eating.

After subsisting on less than 1,000 calories a day for years, binges notwithstanding, I had a friend suggest trying out an at-home fitness streaming service and a portion control-based eating plan.

In this particular portion-controlled nutrition program, color-coded containers corresponded to food groups. There was a list of "approved" foods for each container and, depending on your weight and fitness level, a certain number of each container allotted per day.

Sounded reasonable enough, until I was out of containers and hungry. The feeling of restriction would build and, inevitably, I would binge. It also led to nights with my laptop open, frantically figuring out what I could order on date night with my husband. On those evenings, I should have just ordered what I wanted, what honored my cravings and would leave me feeling satisfied. Instead, I would restrict what I ate during the day to "prepare" for the date night. If that was not possible, I would order not what I truly wanted but what fit into my remaining containers for the day. It also led to me going out with friends armed with containers of food in my purse, eating them when the program said I was supposed to eat.

In all fairness, I will credit this portion-controlled nutrition system for at least getting me one step closer to freedom. At least with the containers, I knew I was eating way more calories than I was before, a number closer to what my body truly needed; but in case you've forgotten, since you've likely been listening to diet culture for too long, *this is still disordered behavior. This is still not freedom.*

I felt trapped in a vicious cycle. Tomorrow, I will be perfect. I will eat perfectly. I will work out perfectly. But when I'd inevitably "mess up," I'd admonish myself. Crawling into bed that night, I would swear to myself that when I woke up the next morning, things would be different—*I* would be different. This went on for years. I was stuck in a cycle that I couldn't break.

I finally had to ask myself: What was this all really about ? Was it really about the weight? The food? My body?

It took me years to discover why the answer was no.

It was about being *in control.* It was about *external validation.* It was about these things that, unbeknownst to me or my well-meaning parents, I thrived on and had been conditioned to seek my entire life; and now that I was an adult, there was no "best" at anything. There was no real A+ or gold star. Life is relative, and as much as I objectively understood that, I couldn't stop those certain neural pathways from firing, driving me to seek perfection, control, and validation.

My recovery, though, led me to the silver lining that is this book and my company. After becoming so passionate about my own recovery and the stories of other women in similar situations, I decided to become a Certified Intuitive Eating Counselor and start Freedom with Food and Fitness at the end of 2020. What better time to create a company, in the middle of a pandemic, when you have a five-month-old son, and just went back to work full-time?

With that said, now might be a proper time for a disclaimer: *Freedom with Food and Fitness* is not intended to be a substitute for professional medical advice, diagnosis, or treatment. Always seek the advice of your physician or another qualified health provider with any questions you may have regarding a medical condition. Never disregard professional medical advice or delay in seeking it because of something you have read in this book. Professional help is *the* most powerful tool for someone seeking mental health awareness or for a disorder.

Why You Need This Book

No matter who you are, you likely wear a lot of hats: mother, father, breadwinner, stay-at-home parent, partner, friend; and no matter what combination of those hats you wear, it's hard work. There's a pressure to do it all, be it all. Some of that pressure comes from society, but a lot of that pressure may also come from yourself in the form of comparison culture. The state of the world makes it difficult to be what society would deem successful, and even when you are, you may harbor guilt for not balancing it all perfectly, all the time.

I know validation and comparison culture are what created my negative relationship with my body. Even though it's been almost a decade since I was in the thick of it, I can remember the shame, the guilt, the frustration, the fear, the brain fog, the lethargy, the worry, the anxiety. I never, ever want another human being to have to feel like that—like they can't trust their own intuition and their own body, like they're not enough for this world and the people in it, that they have to hold themselves to an impossible standard and spend their entire one precious life trying to live up to that standard. It's not fair. It's not right. And it stops here.

I am only one woman, but I am telling my truth in as raw and vulnerable a way as I can in order to give others the strength to take that first step toward recovery and, maybe one day, tell their truth to inspire others, too.

Life is not a zero-sum game. We can all survive, thrive, and lift up those who are still being pushed down and silenced. Am I the supreme expert on eating disorders and intuitive eating? No. Was I sicker than everyone else who has, had, or will have the disorders I did? No. But it was enough to damage my quality of life and open my eyes to the sheer number of people who think, feel, and act the way I did. My lived experience is just as valid as anyone else's, and you should never question if you are "sick enough" to seek help or important enough to tell your truth.

Life happens, and things are out of your control. There may come a time when your resolve weakens and you'll think about going back to your old, disordered ways because they are what you know. It's a familiar devil. Surrounding yourself with like-minded people who speak of food freedom, intuitive eating, and body neutrality will help you remember that this *is* the right path for you. I am fully recovered, but my business forces me to stay immersed in the dialogue and the strategies of this work. I am constantly on Instagram reading what my peers and followers are saying; I'm always listening to podcasts while in the car or doing chores around the house. *Building Freedom with Food and Fitness* keeps me accountable for myself and keeps me conducting myself in a way that I would want my audience to conduct themselves in order to find peace and happiness with their bodies.

So if any part of my story resonates with you, this book is for you. If you've ever looked in the mirror and were disappointed with who you saw looking back at you, this book is for you. If you've ever been fearful or anxious around food, this book is for you. If you've ever felt the pressure to live up to a certain aesthetic in order to be loved, happy, or sexy, this book is for you.

PART 1

Finding Food Freedom

CHAPTER 1

Why We Fall For Diets and Why They Don't Work

In Chapter 4, I will walk you through how to discover *your* reasons for dieting, the pursuit of a different body, and your fraught relationship with food. Once you do a deep dive into your own truth, that truth will set you free; but before I do that, I need to take a few chapters to truly dismantle diet culture and show you why everything you've been told about dieting as it relates to health, self-worth, and happiness is a lie; how most of what you've been told about health and its relation to those things is also a lie. You can't dive into what you truly want when it comes to your body and your health until I reveal those things for what they truly are.

Chances are, if you have been unsatisfied with your body size, you've been on quite a few fad diets, perhaps more than once. In 2020, a survey of 2,000 British citizens found that the average adult will try an average of 126 fad diets over the course of their life; something tells me that number would be much higher if we only looked at women. [3]

---

3. Rebecca Stamp, "Average Person Will Try 126 Fad Diets in Their Lifetime, Poll Claims," *Independent*, January 8, 2020, https://www.independent.co.uk/life-style/diet-weight-loss-food-unhealthy-eating-habits-a9274676.html.

These are called fad diets because they promise fast results and quick fixes to weight and health issues; they are flashes in the cultural pan. Many think their weight loss journey is just about the extra five, ten, twenty pounds they "need to lose," and that once it comes off, they'll be happy, fulfilled, perfect, at peace, whatever it is they're searching to feel. It's not. If you're not addressing the root cause of the issue—your relationship to yourself—you'll gain back that weight once you stop the diet. And you *will* stop the diet, because they are not created to be sustainable long-term.[4] So, you'll have to spend the rest of your life restricting and obsessing about food and weight to maintain your goal. That's not the way I want you to live your life. At that point, is losing the "extra" pounds really worth it?

Why We Fall for Fad Diets

Reason #1: Fad Diets Promote "Clean Slate" and Perfectionist Thinking

We've all seen the commercials: the taut tummies and smiling faces, the dramatic before and after photos, the claims that these diets are easy, fun, "a lifestyle," and "all you have to do is ..." They promise you a new beginning, a transformation. Under the surface are the subliminal, implied messages that you will be more accepted, happier, healthier, more loved, and more confident if you follow these programs. If you have spent years struggling with food and hating your body, that sounds like a pretty good deal. As long as you stick to these

---

4. Traci Mann, A. Janet Tomiyama, Erika Westling, Ann-Marie Lew, Barbra Samuels, and Jason Chatman, "Medicare's Search for Effective Obesity Treatments: Diets Are Not the Answer," *American Psychologist* 62, no. 3 (April 2007): 220–33, https://doi.org/10.1037/0003-066X.62.3.220.

programs, you'll look like the happy, beautiful success stories in the advertisements.

On some level, I think you know it's not true, because the last dozen diets didn't work for you. You couldn't keep up with the exercise program because life happened, you got hungry and ate "off plan," you really wanted that food from that food group you're not supposed to have. These programs are designed in a way that, when you don't get the results you want or stick to the plan, they make you feel that it's your fault you "failed." You beat yourself up because you didn't have the "drive," "determination," or "willpower" to stick with it, forever. I use all these terms in quotation marks because I do not believe these things make a diet successful. So you will try again. And again. And again. Thinking this time, if you just do it perfectly and stay in control, you'll get it right, lose the weight for good, and live happily ever after. This type of thinking leads to a very damaging kind of perfectionism, and the diet industry preys on this. They know perfection is impossible, but thanks to their slick advertising and marketing, you'll keep striving for it. It's genius, really, and the numbers prove it. *Business Wire* reported that the U.S. weight loss and diet control market reached a record $78 billion in 2019.[5]

Clean slate thinking and perfectionism are also super alluring because they give you this dopamine hit in your brain; this intense feeling of reward comes from thinking about the exciting future you've drummed up in your mind, where everything will always be perfect and you will always be happy. When that inevitably doesn't happen,

---

5. "U.S. Weight Loss & Diet Control Market Report 2021: Market Reached a Record $78 Billion in 2019, but Suffered a 21% Decline in 2020 Due to COVID-19 – Forecast to 2025 – ResearchAndMarkets.com," *Business Wire*, March 26, 2021, https://www.businesswire.com/news/home/20210326005126/en/U.S.-Weight-Loss-Diet-Control-Market-Report-2021-Market-Reached-a-Record-78-Billion-in-2019-but-Suffered-a-21-Decline-in-2020-Due-to-COVID-19---Forecast-to-2025---ResearchAndMarkets.com.

you look for that next "high," the next day where you'll be perfect. On and on and on.

For years, I would go to bed at night and consider it to be a reset when my alarm went off the next day. All the mistakes would be erased, including the binges and the foods I "shouldn't" have eaten, and I would be perfect from the moment my alarm went off. It was like *The Truman Show* ... and just as existentially frightening.

It was likely a manifestation of what psychologists call the spotlight effect, where you think people are fixating on you more than they actually are. Society's fixation on aesthetics only serves to fuel this phenomenon which, typically, dissipates in adulthood; but when everywhere you turn you're told to fixate on every pound on your body, you stay perpetually stuck in this self-absorption. Dieting causes you to be, or at least appear to be, preoccupied with how people perceive you, what you look like, etc. It's all very self-centered, as if how your body looks and the number on the scale affects everyone else with whom you interact. You get upset when others don't cater to your dietary needs or when you don't get compliments on the weight you lost. I'm not saying that self-care and prioritizing your needs is a bad thing, but I do take issue with "self-care" when it comes at the expense of others or has its roots in superficial concerns. Again, I am not judging you if you are resonating with these scenarios. These were the cycles I, too, was stuck in and the thoughts that I also had. And let me be the first to tell you that the only way out of them is through a journey that can be messy, shameful, and ugly. The beauty in it, though, is you finally realize that they're simply thoughts, ones you can change with the right strategies.

One strategy to help free yourself here would be to turn your attention outward and cultivate worth that is not tied to your body. You are probably pursuing weight loss or a smaller body because you believe it will bring you happiness or make you worthy, but as it turns out, that's not true; a better route to happiness, according to decades of research, is turning outward and focusing on your connections with others in your life.[6]

When I have a bad body image day, I remember all my contributions to this world that don't have to do with my body. I'm raising an awesome human being, my son Archer, who is 22 months old at the time of this writing. I'm making a difference in the lives of dozens of students, not only by teaching them about literature and journalism, but also by teaching them how to effectively communicate, express themselves, and foster empathy for others.

Contributions aside, realize that you are worthy regardless of those contributions. Everyone is born into this world to serve a purpose. Some will argue that, for example, drug addicts or criminals do not have the same worth as others do, but in fact, they do. Looking at it through a couple of different lenses, they show us the importance of mental health advocacy, or that life is short and to be enjoyed, or that we need to find ways to foster more love in this world to combat the violence and hate. If you disagree, know this is a conscious choice on both of our parts to see the world the way we do. All events and things in life are neutral until you assign meaning to them. I also know everyone is born with worth when I look at my son. He doesn't yet contribute to the world in a way that is traditionally meaningful by adult standards. He does a lot of stuff wrong as he learns to do them right; but he is perfect to me. He is worth more than any aesthetic, success, or wealth I could possibly amass. You, too, were born with that same self-worth.

---

6. Ed Diener and Martin E. P. Seligman, "Very Happy People," *Psychological Science* 13, no. 1 (January 2002): 81–84, https://doi.org/10.1111/1467-9280.00415.

Reason #2: Fad Diets Really Work ... at First

Aside from perfectionist, "clean slate" thinking, another reason you may fall for fad diets is because they work. At first. If you cut carbs from your diet, you *will* see weight loss. What the keto enthusiasts *won't* tell you, though, is that a lot of that initial weight loss is water weight, not fat. When you eat carbs, the energy that you don't use right away is stored as glycogen molecules. Each gram of glycogen comes with three grams of water attached.[7] So in those first two weeks, the dramatic weight loss you're seeing is water. The keto diet isn't some magic solution to your weight woes. In fact, the keto diet was originally introduced by physicians as a way to treat childhood epilepsy in the 1920s.[8] It's also not sustainable. Are you really going to follow a diet that limits your carbs, *even your fruit intake*, for *the rest of your life*? Really, think about that. It's not healing your relationship with food by teaching you to fear it. It's not healing your relationship with your body either, only manipulating your body, and probably in a way it doesn't want to be.

An article in *Medical News Today* reported that "weight loss plateaus happen after about six months of following a low calorie diet. Doctors are unsure why weight loss plateaus occur, but some theories include: the body adapts to weight loss and *defends itself against further weight loss* [emphasis added]."[9] Shouldn't that be a signal to stop dieting? If the body has to protect itself from further weight loss,

7. Valentín E. Fernández-Elías, Juan F. Ortega, Rachael K. Nelson, and Ricardo Mora-Rodriguez, "Relationship between Muscle Water and Glycogen Recovery after Prolonged Exercise in the Heat in Humans," *European Journal of Applied Physiology* 115, no. 9 (September 2015): 1919–26, https://doi.org/10.1007/s00421-015-3175-z.

8. James W. Wheless, "History of the Ketogenic Diet," *Epilepsia* 49, suppl. 8 (November 2008): 3–5, https://doi.org/10.1111/j.1528-1167.2008.01821.x.

9. Jessica Caporuscio, "What to Do About a Weight Loss Plateau," *Medical News Today*, September 23, 2019, https://www.medicalnewstoday.com/articles/326415.

because it thinks it's experiencing a famine, doesn't that say to you that losing any more weight for your particular body is unhealthy?

If the way you've been eating feels sustainable long-term to you, a plateau can actually be a wonderful thing. Perhaps you've reached your weight set range! Your weight set range is the body weight range that your genetics have determined is ideal for your specific body. [10] Everyone has a different weight set range, even if you're the same height or age. Discovering your weight set range should be celebrated because you're honoring your body's genetic blueprint. The diet and fitness industries, however, want you to see a plateau as a sign of failure because, if we successfully reach our weight set range, then we don't need them anymore; but really, our bodies have reached their destinations! It's all maintenance and listening to our bodies from then on out.

Looking a certain way doesn't heal your relationship with your body because what happens if you can't look that way anymore? And trust me, you won't forever, anyway. You will age, your skin will sag, your metabolism will slow; and so will mine and everyone around us. If you can't love yourself now, what makes you think you'll love yourself then? In order to have long-term satisfaction with your body, you need to stop moralizing food as good or bad and cultivate self-worth, regardless of what you look like. That's why you should try journaling and reflecting on how else you provide value to this world: you cultivate a sense of compassion and love for yourself and those around you that supersedes the "shell" you live in.

Maybe you're thinking that's unfair. It's easy for me, as a thin person, to say, "Yeah, well, not everyone gets to be thin." I sympathize with this because I recognize that there are particular hardships

---

10. Manfred J. Müller, Anya Bosy-Westphal, and Steven B. Heymsfield, "Is There Evidence for a Set Point that Regulates Human Body Weight?" *F1000 Medicine Reports* 2, no. 59 (August 2010): 1–7, https://doi.org/10.3410/M2-59.

that larger-bodied individuals face in this thin-obsessed society that I will never understand firsthand. Stigma, prejudice, and discrimination against those in larger bodies is not only a real but also a prevalent reality to contend with, from airplane seats to quality healthcare. What I can offer is the aforementioned perspective that every thought you have is a choice. You can choose to embrace your body as it is and call a truce to the war with yourself. The only alternative is to fight against your own reality, and in that fight, you will always lose. Heck, try even showing those who stigmatize you some compassion. If they are that ingrained in fatphobia, they are already probably punishing themselves, too. They haven't been enlightened the way you have, and that's a shame.

Reason #3: Fad Diets Hijack Body Trust and We Become Reliant on Them

You might not remember it, but when you were a baby, you were offered food. If you were hungry, you ate it. If you weren't hungry, you'd push it away; or in my son's case, throw it on the floor, and let's be honest, sometimes at me. It was as simple as that. You listened to and trusted your body to know exactly what kind of food you wanted and how much. Somewhere along the way, you learned that certain foods were "good" and "healthy" and other foods were "bad" and "unhealthy." And like anything else, when we're told something that seems attractive should be avoided, we gravitate toward it. Humans, by nature, are hardwired to test limits and rebel to find where "the line" is. I believe this is the foundation of the "terrible twos" we're currently experiencing in this household.

As a child, you were told, either explicitly or inferentially, that thin bodies are the ideal and that body fat is to be avoided at all costs. Perhaps you were told that people in larger bodies are lazy or lack willpower and self-control. Maybe you saw classmates in larger bodies being bullied at school, and you didn't want to be bullied, so you attempted to avoid getting bigger yourself. If your parents brought you to the doctor and you weighed more than you "should," your doctor—whom the whole family considered a health expert—may have told you that you needed to be put on a diet: cut sugar, cut carbs, cut calories.

This fatphobic, lazy, knee-jerk prescription to shrink larger bodies, which is what we should *actually* fear, creates an underlying narrative: people in larger bodies are "less than." People in larger bodies need to change. And this narrative is created at a startlingly early age.

For those of you who have kids, although you can't stop others from broadcasting these narratives, whether they're explicit or inferred, you can filter them in our own home. Read books to your children that include characters of all body types, and while you're at it, skin colors, abilities, etc. Be mindful of your language when talking about your own body or the bodies of others, whether they be real people or characters on TV. Be conscious of not only your narratives but also your behaviors such as body checking, which includes constantly checking the mirror, pinching fat, etc. Offer your children a variety of foods. Do not force them to finish what's on their plate, but instead, ask them to ask their tummies how they feel. Are they still hungry or full? Ask them questions about their foods as they eat to promote mindful eating. Where do they think eggs come from? What color are they? Are they hot or cold? How does the texture feel in their mouths? Don't glorify "healthier" foods or praise your children for eating them. All foods should remain neutral with no moral value attached to them. Sometimes, all my two-year-old son Archer wants for dinner is tortilla chips, or as he calls them, "crackers." Other times, he'll eat a salmon burger and mixed vegetables. I don't push the latter on him because my only job is to offer the food options to him, and he chooses what he wants and in the amount he wants. That is the very definition of intuitive eating.

Bodies are very smart and we should trust them. Your child's body will naturally crave a variety of foods without you having to coax them into it. When you're craving meat, for example, it is likely your body is in need of iron. Those who crave fatty foods might not be getting enough calcium. Your children won't starve. As most parents know, the second you try to force anything onto your kids is the second they don't want those things anyway!

Reason #4: Fad Diets Undermine the Very Things You Need to Be Authentically Healthy in the First Place: Self-Confidence and Self-Acceptance

Companies who push fad diets aren't stupid; they know which marketing strategies are effective. They know how to provide testimonials from real customers, although these testimonials are probably done during the initial "miracle" weight loss phase. They know to use the following buzz words: easy, fun, strong, wellness, healthy, lifestyle, and happy.

Their marketing is done in a way that makes you feel that *when*, not if, the diet doesn't provide the desired result, it's your fault. Something must be wrong with you. You must be weak-willed. You must not want it enough. Because nothing tastes as good as skinny feels, right?

So you keep trying, either the same diet or a new one that shows promise of a life where you love yourself in your new, skinny body. And you inevitably keep failing, each time chipping more and more away from your self-esteem, self-confidence, and self-love, if you even had any to begin with. The most famous statistic against weight loss and diets is that ninety-five percent of diets fail and most people will regain their lost weight within one to five years.[11] It can't be that nine-ty-five percent of people are weak-willed. Just like when you have that girlfriend who can't seem to make any of her relationships work, at some point, you kind of want to ask her if she's ever wondered if it's her, not them.

These other people in the commercial did it; why can't I? My college roommate lost all that weight and looks great in a bikini at the beach with her family. Why can't I?

The reality is that you have no idea what it really took for someone to achieve the desired aesthetic. You don't know their genetics, how often they work out, how much or little they eat, whether they purge or exhibit any other disordered behaviors like taking fat burners. Even if some Instagram fitness influencer posts "what I eat in a day," you don't know how accurate that is. Sure, she might eat it, but the whole thing? Does she throw it back up? Will she fast the entire day tomorrow? Or spend four hours at the gym working it off? You just don't know. So to compare anyone else's journey or body to our own is futile because there are too many, often hidden, variables. All of the times someone told me I looked great or skinny when I was sick, I just said, "Thank you." What I really wanted to do was be honest, put down the armor of perfection, and tell someone what I was experiencing, to reach out for help.

Although there were many factors that contributed to my eating disorders, the event that actually set the wheels in motion, I'm embarrassed to say, was a negligible one. I saw a picture of my then boyfriend's ex-girlfriend at the beach. I had always been self-conscious about my lack of visible abdominals. I don't remember how it came up, but he mentioned her weight to me, and it was a few pounds less

11. Albert Stunkard and Mavis McLaren-Hume, "The Results of Treatment for Obesity: A Review of the Literature and Report of a Series," AMA Archives of Internal Medicine 103, no. 1 (January 1959): 79–85, https://doi.org/10.1001/archinte.1959.00270010085011.

than what I weighed at the time. So, I wanted to weigh less than her. Because I wanted to feel the "best" at something, at a time in my life where I felt I couldn't measure my own worth with grades anymore, and at the time, I thought "skinny" was synonymous with "best."

Never mind that I had no idea if she worked out, what she ate, how much, whether she was disordered, or what her genetics were. Never mind the fact that my boyfriend was with me and not with her for reasons that, I can only assume, weren't related to our respective bodies.

The more you try to manipulate your body and compare your body to other people's, the more you are internalizing this narrative that we are not enough just as we are, the more you are perpetuating the cultural narrative that thin is best. That something with you is broken and needs to be fixed, and that's just not the case. Dieting companies don't sell you change because they altruistically want you to be a better version of yourself; they care about their profit margins.

Diets: The Short-Term Band-Aid for the Long-Term Bullet Wound

The statistics and studies that prove diets don't work are very accessible online; whether you'll see them in mainstream media is another story. "Wellness" businesses thrive on the idea that diets work and count on the fact that you're unhappy with your body. If they didn't and you weren't, they'd be out of business.

Let's go back to that "ninety-five percent of diets fail" statistic. According to a more recent *New York Times* article, that study was very small, and therefore, perhaps not the most valid. [12] The article itself,

---

12. Jane Fritsch, "95% Regain Lost Weight. Or Do They?" *New York Times*, May 25, 1999, F7, http://www.nytimes.com/1999/05/25/health/95-regain-lost-weight-or-do-they.html.

however, has wording I would like to challenge. The piece ends with a quote from a source: "'You just have to change your lifestyle,' he said. 'You just have to have the willpower to do it.' But that is not necessarily easy,' he conceded. 'You just have to weigh the choices. Do you want to become healthier?'"

My issue with that quote is that *weight loss and health are not the same thing*. When I was sick, I vacillated between what would be considered normal weight and underweight. My mind and my body were desperate for love, control, safety, and validation. I was so preoccupied with when I could eat and all the food I wasn't allowing myself that I would, very frequently, and quite literally, dream of food several nights a week. I was happy when I woke up that I enjoyed the food in my sleep but didn't have to worry about the real-life calorie repercussions of eating the dream food. That's not mental health; that's mental illness.

Whether the original "ninety-five percent" study is valid or not doesn't really matter. Maybe most people can't be consistent with their diets because they're unsustainable. Maybe some people can lose weight and keep it off because they become accustomed to a certain way of eating that doesn't feel restrictive; but the point is if you're approaching your eating and fitness *from a place of wanting to change your body because you're unhappy with who you are*, no diet will ever fix that. You're looking to put on a topical cream when you really need an oral medication, trying to fix something you believe is on the surface when it's really systemic. If you're administering treatment, no amount of that treatment will fix the ailment, both literally and figuratively.

In fact, healing your insides will actually help "heal" your outsides, not the other way around. An article in the *Psychotherapy Networker* found that being in a body larger than your genetic weight set range may be the result of early life trauma. In one study of 286 people categorized as "obese," half had been sexually abused as children. In these cases, "overeating and obesity weren't the central problems, but attempted solutions." [13] A much larger study of more than 17,000 people provided further documentation of the links between "adverse childhood experiences" and unhealthy behaviors like smoking, drinking, and overeating.

Usually diet culture burrows into people's minds for one of two reasons: culture/society has drilled it into them or they've experienced some sort of trauma. In the case of those who were sexually abused, eating may have become a coping mechanism for feelings of shame, fear, and anxiety. While it's okay to have an occasional rough day at work and intentionally decide to mindfully have some cookies, it's another to use overeating as a long-term crutch for an issue that requires therapy and deep emotional and mental healing. More about the potential deeper reasons behind your broken relationship with food and your body in the next chapter.

If there was one way to eat for optimal health, there wouldn't be keto, which praises fats; or low-fat diets, which obviously don't work. A few years ago, nutritionists were saying eggs were good for us, then they were bad, then only the whites were good, and now it's the whole egg; if you're a fan of standup comedy, I highly recommend Lewis Black's skit on this. In the '90s, the "Got Milk?" campaign was huge, and now studies show that drinking cow's milk may actually be detrimental to bone health and be linked to prostate and ovarian cancers. [14] My point here is not to make you afraid of food; I feed my son whole eggs and whole milk, regardless of the studies, because I don't buy too

13. Meg Selig, "Why Diets Don't Work ... and What Does," *Psychology Today*, October 21, 2010, http://www.psychologytoday.com/us/blog/changepower/201010/why-diets-dont-work-and-what-does.

14. Sencer, "Is Milk Good or Bad for You?" *KQED*, March 9, 2016, http://www.kqed.org/education/130193/is-milk-good-or-bad-for-you.

much into the hype of either camp; and that's because it seems as if, for all our scientific studies and research, there is no definitive information regarding different food groups and their role in our health and longevity. Our knowledge of foods and nutrition is constantly evolving and largely depending on who is eating them. We should also be skeptical regarding the validity and objectivity of studies, because many times, studies will come to a conclusion that just so happens to benefit the organization that funded the study.

So you have to ask: What are you really searching for? It might be control, external validation, attractiveness in the eyes of society, or to just be someone different because you don't like who you are. What are you really looking to heal? Is it your relationship with yourself or a trauma you've experienced that you need to process and release? You need to find the answers to those questions, and do some deep reflecting and healing; and in the meantime, eat what feels good in your body. Eat in an amount that leaves you feeling nourished and satiated.

CHAPTER 2

Underlying Reasons You May Have Issues with Food and Your Body

I can't tell you how many women think they have issues with food. They believe they can't be trusted around it, that they have some sort of addiction to it. I know better than to never say never, but I would say only in very rare cases are people actually addicted to food. A 2013 study showed that only 5.4% (6.7% in females and 3.0% in males) of the people in the study were actually addicted to food; and I would wager that many of these "addicted" people are addicted due to restriction.[15] The fact that the study showed an increase in food addiction for those labeled as obese, again, probably speaks to the power of binge—restrict cycles to slow metabolism, raise the body's natural weight range, and therefore, increase people's weight.

One of the biggest epiphanies I had in my journey to food freedom was realizing that my issues were never about the food. It was

---

15. Pardis Pedram, Danny Wadden, Peyvand Amini, Wayne Gulliver, Edward Randell, et al., "Food Addiction: Its Prevalence and Significant Association with Obesity in the General Population," *PLOS ONE* 8, no. 9 (September 2013): 1–6, https://doi.org/10.1371/journal.pone.0074832.

a combination of the desire for control, perfectionism, external validation, and people pleasing that I spoke about in the introduction. Those came together to manifest their desires in a trove of eating disorders and disordered eating behaviors. In the same way, if you peel back the layers of what you're experiencing with food and your body, chances are you will find a larger, underlying issue masking itself as disordered eating, poor body image, chronic dieting, etc.

Big "T" and Little "T" Trauma

Trauma can be a reason for one's damaged relationship with food and body. Typically these traumas occur when you are a child, in your formative years, when your brain and beliefs about yourself and the world are still developing. They are events that can shape the very way you see the world, yourself, and other people. Because they tend to be ingrained within your psyche as truth over time, these harmful narratives are particularly difficult to erase.

You may be thinking this doesn't apply to you, but there are two different kinds of trauma: Big "T" Trauma and Little "T" Trauma. Big "T" traumas are, as the name suggests, larger traumas that cause Post Traumatic Stress Disorder (PTSD). In fact, about one-third of women with bulimia, twenty percent with binge eating disorder, and 11.8% with non-bulimic/non-binge eating disorders met criteria for lifetime PTSD.[16] Traumas that result in PTSD can include sexual abuse, chronic or intense physical abuse, witnessing the untimely death of a loved one, or life-threatening experiences. On the other hand, many more of us have experienced Little "T" Traumas: forms of bullying, watching loved ones dieting, or some other type of

---

16. Timothy D. Brewerton, "Eating Disorders, Trauma, and Comorbidity: Focus on PTSD," *Eating Disorders* 15, no. 4 (August 2007): 285–304, https://doi.org/10.1080/10640260701454311.

emotional damage. It's worth noting, too, that Little "T" Traumas are just as valid, and those who are affected by Little "T" Traumas have just as much of a right to seek professional help as those who experience Big "T" Traumas. Although not divided into Big "T" and Little "T" traumas, the U.S. Department of Veteran Affairs reported that sixty percent of men and fifty percent of women experience at least one trauma in their lives, with women more likely to experience sexual assault and child sexual abuse.[17]

Two anecdotal, albeit very similar, stories of how trauma can manifest itself into an eating disorder show how, more likely than not, your issues with food aren't actually about the food. In one woman's experience, she had been raped as a little girl and, as an adult, tried to make herself as big as possible with food so that no other man would see her as attractive and try to sexually assault her. Another woman did the opposite: She tried to shrink her body as much as she possibly could, almost as a way to make herself invisible to men, after being sexually assaulted by her father as a young girl.

As is the case with these two women, they tried to control their bodies in order to protect themselves from the kind of harm they endured in their formative years. Instead of living for pleasure, their modus operandi was minimizing pain. Controlling their bodies was their default defense mechanism to cope with their pasts.

Perfectionism and Defending Yourself Against Criticism

There are three types of perfectionism. Socially-prescribed perfectionism comes from the crippling fear of criticism; basically, the belief that if someone is not the best, they will be rejected by those around them,

---

17. "How Common Is PTSD in Adults?" National Center for PTSD, U.S. Department of Veterans Affairs, last modified April 8, 2022, http://www.ptsd.va.gov/understand/common/common_adults.asp.

including loved ones. This can lead to procrastination because they fear doing something wrong. Other-oriented perfectionists put impossibly high standards on others, instead of themselves. Self-oriented perfectionists are those who place these high standards on themselves, but unlike those who suffer from socially-prescribed perfectionism, they can achieve goals, albeit never as perfectly as they would want to.

I undoubtedly fell into the last category. When I messed up or didn't "perform" up to my own unrealistically high standards, I would shame myself for not being perfect and feel the overwhelming compulsion to "start over" the next day. This cycle went on for years, and dare I admit, decades. I never allowed myself any of the grace or self-compassion I would freely give to others. I achieved a lot in my life, but it was never enough, and the painfully ironic thing was, many of my larger achievements felt empty because I got more pleasure out of the striving than the end result.

The pressure to be perfect led me to want to weigh the perfect amount, eat the perfect amount, and have the perfect body. That type of restriction, naturally, led to binge eating and feeling out of control with food. Remember, if you go against what your body needs to function properly, it will inevitably rebel against what you want, despite any "willpower" or white-knuckling you try to exhibit.

I'm certainly not the only one to experience this—and it's getting worse. In a 2017 study in *Psychological Bulletin*, researchers evaluated more than 40,000 college students in the U.S., Canada, and the UK between 1989 and 2016. Over the course of those twenty-seven years, perfectionistic tendencies increased across the board, with socially-prescribed perfectionism rising at the greatest rate, thirty-two percent.[18]

Why do perfectionists act the way they do? Much of the time, it's for a similar reason as the two women who controlled their bodies as

18. Thomas Curran and Andrew P. Hill, "Perfectionism Is Increasing over Time: A Meta-analysis of Birth Cohort Differences from 1989 to 2016," *Psychological Bulletin* 145, no. 4 (2019): 410–29, https://doi.org/10.1037/bul0000138.

a way to protect themselves from future sexual abuse: They try to protect themselves from criticism and minimize pain, which were my motivations as a perfectionist. If I could just be perfect, no one would say anything bad about me. If I was thin, I would be beautiful, and I would receive praise instead of criticism. It was a defense mechanism for low intrinsic self-worth, which later became an issue in adulthood when there is no best at anything. I was afraid of being stripped of that title in all areas of my life as my world expanded after college, so I clung to things I thought I could control: my weight and my food.

As we've seen, though, you can't *really* control your weight; it is, more or less, biologically determined;[19] and anything you do to control it will only trigger a lifelong battle with your body and your mind.

Validation and Low Self-Worth

Validation played a huge part in my eating disorder. It was like a drug for me. The more people affirmed that I was smart or beautiful or whatever, the more I craved it. It made me feel worthy. It made me feel valuable. And when you feed on external validation, you never learn how to cultivate inner validation. I never had to rely on it.

I know how that sounds. Oh, poor me. Compliments abound. Of course, it's nice to get compliments, and I could consider myself lucky to have the conventional traits that garner such compliments, but in the long run, it really did me more harm than good.

There's a twofold solution to healing from this validation addiction: 1) learn how to cultivate internal validation and 2) stop relying on external validation. Intrinsic validation requires the belief that—no

---

19. "Why People Become Overweight," *Harvard Health Publishing*, June 24, 2019, https://www.health.harvard.edu/staying-healthy/why-people-become-overweight.

matter what you look like, your successes, your failures, etc.—you are worthy of the life you want to live. As I said in the previous chapter, we are all born into this life and deserve a place in it. Life is a precious and fragile miracle, and by extension, we're all precious and fragile miracles and should treat ourselves as such.

Cultivating internal validation requires us to stop worrying about what other people think and comparing ourselves to others. In fact, a study in the *Journal of Personality and Social Psychology* concluded that intrinsic motivation helped to combat comparison culture.[20] We can't find ourselves to be intrinsically worthy if we're always measuring ourselves against others and their unique worthiness. Weight, careers, children, bodies, money—they're not meant to be compared because there are so many variables in everyone's lives that it's not fair or even logical to compare in terms of "the best." That's a lesson I had to learn the hard way.

Who you want validation from also matters in terms of figuring out our why. Is it a male figure in your life, if you're someone who identifies as a heterosexual female? Or men in general? Perhaps you need to look into your childhood and adult relationship with your father, or lack thereof. What about your mother? What type of relationship did she have with your father or, if she is/was divorced, with other men? For example, if you saw your mother constantly try to seek validation from the men she dated through the way she looked, you probably look for the same validation through the way you look. If your parents only showed you love and affection when you were successful, that can set you up to seek external validation, too.

There are many ways to cultivate internal validation, and they all begin in the mind; there's so much, in fact, that I could write a whole

---

20. Jeff Schimel, Jamie Arndt, Tom Pyszczynski, and Jeff Greenberg, "Being Accepted for Who We Are: Evidence that Social Validation of the Intrinsic Self Reduces General Defensiveness," *Journal of Personality and Social Psychology* 80, no. 1 (January 2001): 35–52, https://doi.org/10.1037//0022-3514.80.1.35.

other book about it. Since you're reading *this* book, though, some things to consider would be how you speak to yourself. When you complete a goal, are you congratulating yourself in a compassionate way, instead of looking for other people to do it for you? Are *you* proud of yourself? Many find that inner child work, where you visualize yourself as a child, makes it easier to show yourself self-compassion and love.

Other people's validation is really more about them and what they value and find to be worthy. Everyone else's opinions about the world and about us are simply a reflection of their own minds and beliefs about themselves. Furthermore, their approval is conditional; it only lasts as long as you do things that please them. This people-pleasing mentality will only serve to set you up for a life that is lived for everyone else but you. And lastly, doing things in your life that are in line with your own values and beliefs will help you cultivate internal validation. What is important to you? How do you want to show up in the world? Because there will always be a critic, someone who thinks you're too much of this and not enough of that. You will never please all of them. There is quite literally no one else in the world like you, and in order to do what you were meant to in this world, while staying in integrity with your beliefs, you need to do those things for yourself and be your biggest cheerleader along the way.

Mental Illness

There are several mental illnesses that can contribute to or manifest as eating disorders. For example, people who suffer from depression tend to feel unworthy or broken. This could lead to an attempt to "fix" themselves through disordered dieting and exercise. They are trying to conventionally fit into society's version of who is worthy, thanks to diet culture. A 1990 study in *Behaviour Research and Therapy* found that the "thin ideal," the socially prescribed idea that the ideal body is thin and small, causes depression at a higher rate among women than among men. [21]

Unfortunately, the symptoms of depression typically only worsen once an eating disorder is present. Loss of appetite, lack of sleep, feelings of hopelessness, loss of sex drive, and feelings of sadness become elevated with an eating disorder, and the cycle continues.

Anxiety, and in particular obsessive—compulsive disorder (OCD), can also go hand-in-hand with eating disorders. I experienced this with body dysmorphic disorder (BDD). BDD is a subset of OCD where you have a constant preoccupation with a particular body part's perceived flaw; typically, that flaw is very minor or possibly not even there at all. We must also keep in mind that the word "flaw" is subjective. I constantly felt the compulsion to check my stomach in the mirror. Objectively, I knew that it was impossible that my stomach had, all of a sudden, drastically changed from one hour to the next, but I couldn't stop myself from checking, almost as a way to reassure myself, "You're still 'fit.' Therefore, you're still 'safe.'" It would drive me insane some days because the more I looked, the more I wanted to keep looking, and it became a cycle I couldn't break. I can't tell you how many collective hours I wasted doing this. According to a 2004 study in *World Psychiatry*, BDD steals an average of three to eight hours per day from a person who suffers with it. [22]

These are not the only underlying reasons you may have a broken relationship with food and your body. Everyone's situation is different and nuanced, and so is this work of finding freedom. Working with a therapist, dietitian, or Certified Intuitive Eating Counselor can help you dig deeper into your specific needs.

---

21. Mandy McCarthy, "The Thin Ideal, Depression and Eating Disorders in Women," *Behaviour Research and Therapy* 28, no. 3 (1990): 205–14, https://doi.org/10.1016/0005-7967(90)90003-2.

22. Katharine A. Phillips, "Body Dysmorphic Disorder: Recognizing and Treating Imagined Ugliness," *World Psychiatry* 3, no. 1 (February 2004): 12–17.

CHAPTER 3

Replacing Counting and Weighing with Body Trust

Trigger warning: I use numbers for calories, macros, and weight in this chapter to prove a point about how they are not to be trusted.

There is only one time that I would suggest calorie counting, macro counting, or a body weight scale to anyone, and that's if they are in an active eating disorder where there is heavy restriction. When someone enters treatment for recovery from a disorder like anorexia nervosa, there is a refeeding period, where caloric intake is increased with the help of a professional, after a period of little to no food intake. Structured meal times and meal plans may be utilized. If this is you and you feel this is what you need as your next step of recovery, intuitive eating may not be an appropriate step for you right now. I would highly suggest seeking the help of an eating disorder treatment center or a registered non-diet dietitian.

Why Online Calculators Cannot Be Trusted

In order to write this chapter, I consulted about ten online calculators that promised to tell me my caloric range. One online calculator that I chose at random on the Internet told me that my basal metabolic rate (BMR) is 1,279 calories. BMR is how many calories you need to consume in order to simply survive, if your body is at rest. That's not factoring in any physical activity that I do throughout the day or my particular genetics.

Another website told me my BMR was 1,340 calories, and another said 1,451 calories.

First of all, 1,200 calories a day is considered starvation, so I'm definitely not eating only 1,279 calories a day. In fact, the typical two-year-old requires 1,000 to 1,400 calories a day. So if you've been eating less than what these calculators have been suggesting for you, you've *really* been depriving your body of calories. In starvation mode, your body will *hold onto* calories and fat, by slowing down your metabolism, in an attempt to survive. It's a biological response from when we were hunters and gatherers who didn't know when our next meal was coming. If your body doesn't trust you to feed it, it's going to do everything it can to stay alive. A slow metabolism means fewer calories and less fat burned throughout the day. Not only that, you can actually *raise* your weight set range, not lower it, by dieting.[23] Some researchers believe that with chronic dieting, leptin and insulin resistance develops, which causes us to gain weight.[24] Funny how diet culture conveniently leaves that part out when it preaches that you should be eating at a massive calorie deficit to see results!

---

23. Mann, et al., "Medicare's Search."

24. Chang Hee Jung and Min-Seon Kim, "Molecular Mechanisms of Central Leptin Resistance in Obesity," *Archives of Pharmacal Research* 36, no. 2 (January 2013): 201–207, https://doi.org/10.1007/s12272-013-0020-y.

Secondly, let's talk about how much these numbers differ! Who is to say that the calculator you used to get the number of calories you're allowing yourself per day is even accurate? These calculators are fallible computer programs. You're letting some random calculator on some random dude's fitness website dictate whether you feel guilty for the rest of the day for eating an extra snack or second helping of dinner because you were trying to honor your hunger. Does that sound rational? When it comes down to it, these calculators and even personal trainers who tell you calorie limits don't know your body's personal needs; only your body knows those.

So, taking the largest number of the three, am I going to 1,451 calories a day? Nope. Again, these numbers don't account for physical activity throughout the day. I work out six days a week and carry around and chase around my very active son. We take walks after dinner with the stroller. I'm up and down stairs at work. And every day is different! Some days, I'm more active than others. So rigidly following a calorie limit and struggling to remain inside the parameters of that limit every day is unnecessary and damaging. I have a general idea, from all my years of dieting, of how many calories will leave me feeling my best throughout the day, but I no longer count them. I've arrived at my weight set range and maintaining it is effortless.

You will know when you've arrived at your weight set range if you can, more often than not, identify and honor your hunger, fullness, and satiety cues; I say "more often than not" because we're only human, and sometimes even a veteran intuitive eater can over or undereat; the key, though, is they don't make it mean anything about them or their self-worth. You'll also know if you're eating an adequate amount of food each day if your weight remains relatively stable. Although I wouldn't recommend weighing yourself, you will notice the way your clothes fit you stays consistent. You will likely also notice a marked improvement in your mental clarity, disposition, sleep, and physical energy.

Why Scales Cannot Be Trusted

Since we were young enough to visit a pediatrician, we've heard about BMI, body mass index. This is a number that is determined with your height, sex, and weight, which categorizes you as underweight, normal, overweight, or obsese.

Let me be blunt in saying that BMI is medically invalid in many cases. Its inventor, Adolphe Quetelet, originally created the BMI scale as a way to measure populations of people, not as a barometer of someone's individual health. In fact, weight wasn't considered a barometer of health until the twentieth century, when life insurance companies started using it as a way to increase customer premiums. Then, in 1998, the U.S. National Institutes of Health and the Centers for Disease Control and Prevention lowered the normal/overweight threshold from a BMI of 27.8 to 25. Clearly, what's considered normal weight versus overweight isn't an absolute truth if they can simply change the ranges.

During much of my eating disorder, I fell within the normal weight category, but it wasn't where *my* body wanted to be. That weight may have been fine for another woman of my age and height, but my body's genetic blueprint said otherwise for me; and my body let me know it was pissed. I was tired all the time, I found it very hard to concentrate, and I was irritable much of the time because I was chronically ignoring my hunger.

Just as you can be unhealthy, as I was, at a "normal" BMI weight, you can also be healthy outside of it. I have known plenty of people in larger bodies who are in shape, feel good in their bodies, and have exceptional blood work results. In a 2008 peer-reviewed study, a team of doctors concluded: "Despite the good correlation between BMI and BF% [body fat percentage], the diagnostic accuracy of BMI to diagnose obesity is limited, particularly for individuals in the intermediate BMI ranges." [25] The definition of obesity is a disorder involving excessive body fat that increases the risk of health problems. So, by definition, obesity isn't about body weight, *per se*, but body fat. So then if we have a "better" indicator of health than weight-to-height ratios (BMI) by assessing body fat percentages, why aren't we using that? Because accurately measuring body fat percentages is more difficult, invasive, and costly. The medical community only continues to use BMI because it's easier and cheaper to use in categorizing people as obese, not because it's particularly accurate at measuring health.

I'm not proposing we start measuring body fat in lieu of body weight. Focusing on body fat and losing it only potentially puts a Band-Aid on a bullet wound. If you're carrying around excess body fat, there are issues like anxiety, depression, lack of coping mechanisms, emotional management, self-care, and self-worth that need to be attended to, not the body fat itself. A restrictive diet will not fix those things, and on the other hand, some people just have more body fat than others naturally. And that's okay, too. The reference of body fat being a more accurate indicator of health is only to point out that doctors are simply using BMI because it's more convenient for them, not because it is a better quality assessment of health.

Let me reiterate that *any weight, in and of itself, is not bad or unhealthy*. There's no moral attachment to weight, which is what

---

25. Abel Romero-Corral, Virend K. Somers, Justo Sierra-Johnson, Randal J. Thomas, Kent R. Bailey, Maria L. Collazo-Clavell, Thomas G. Allison, Josef Korinek, John A. Batsis, F. H. Sert-Kuniyoshi, and Francisco Lopez-Jimenez, "Accuracy of Body Mass Index in Diagnosing Obesity in the Adult General Population," *International Journal of Obesity* 32, no. 6 (July 2008): 959–66, https://doi.org/10.1038/ijo.2008.11.

those who advocate for Health at Every Size (HAES) believe. *If you have a loving relationship with food and your body,* whatever weight you are at is right for you. If you have a sense of self-worth and know how to manage your thoughts and emotions, you can be healthy in a small body or a larger one. That being said, it's worth mentioning that the term is Health at Every Size, not *Healthy* at Every Size. People of any size can participate in healthful behaviors, but I would find it hard to believe someone who weighs 600 pounds is healthy. Someone that far out of the typical weight range for their age and height probably has an underlying medical issue or is using food as some sort of coping mechanism for emotions or trauma.

Why Macro Counting Cannot Be Trusted, but We Still Need Macronutrients

Lastly for this chapter, let's look at macronutrient, or "macro," counting. I tried this after I decided the containers were too restrictive for me. I loved the allure of the "if it fits in your macros." *Finally, food freedom!* I thought. I can have wine and cheese and pizza without feeling guilty, so long as it fits in my allotted macros!

For those who don't know what macros are and how one counts them, let me break it down for you quickly. There are three types of macronutrients your body needs: fat, carbohydrates, and protein. Those who follow diets based on macros believe that the body functions optimally when we eat a certain amount of grams of each macronutrient or a certain percentage of each. For example, the macro percentages for someone looking to gain muscle is approximately forty percent protein, thirty percent fat, and thirty percent carbs. Depending on your weight and calorie limit, that will equate to a certain amount of grams of each per day. Tracking apps provide ways to track these numbers throughout your day.

Here's where things get disordered. What if, say, at the end of the day, you're craving an apple as a snack, but you've already eaten your allotted carbs for the day? Do you not honor that craving, even though an apple is nutrient-dense and delicious? Do you reach for a hard boiled egg, even though that's not what you want, because it fits better into your macros? By doing this, you're denying yourself what you truly want, which will likely result in a binge later. You'll be full, but not satiated. Also, that hard boiled egg has both protein *and* fat. Having that egg will get you to your protein goal for the day, but then put you over your allotted fats for the day.

See what I mean? All this tracking and manipulation can drive a person crazy.

I do, however, think the *idea* of macros can be useful. We know that we need to have some of each macronutrient throughout the day. I keep that in the back of my mind throughout the day as I choose things to eat. If I notice I haven't had much fat throughout the day, I try to choose something for dinner or my nighttime snack that includes fats, but I won't choose something I don't genuinely want. Luckily, there are plenty of foods with fats in them, so it's typically not difficult. And hello, who doesn't like peanut butter, avocado, or chocolate?

Conversely, if I know that I'm having carb- or fat-dense foods at night for a date night or holiday party, I will try to find protein sources earlier in the day that sound yummy to me. If I truly can't find one and all I want for breakfast is toast with jelly, then I honor that, but usually when I run through the list of things I could have for breakfast that include protein, I can find something that strikes my fancy that I'll truly enjoy and will leave my body feeling good afterward. This is also part of what intuitive eaters mean by gentle nutrition. We are, contrary to popular belief, thinking about nutrition and nutrient-dense foods so our bodies feel good.

I try to incorporate a mix of fats, proteins, and carbs into all my meals. If I'm craving a salad and throw in lettuce, veggies, and chicken, I'll stop and ask myself if there's a fat I'm craving that would go well in the salad. Sometimes it's avocado, sometimes it's cheese. Sometimes a scoop of peanut butter on the side sounds good to me, as weird as that sounds, so that's what I go with. If I truly don't want to add anything more to the salad or on the side, then I don't, but I always ask myself if there's a way I can incorporate all three macronutrients into my meal. This creates a meal with "staying power," by providing sustained energy and stabilizing blood-glucose levels. There's no weighing, measuring, or counting, though; I just add what sounds good to me in the moment, keeping in mind how my body will feel afterward, as well.

Body weight, calories, and macronutrients should never be things that you let determine your day: emotionally, mentally, or behaviorally. Once that happens, you let diet culture rule your life, and you need to revisit your why. Life is about moments and memories, not macros. If you're missing out on opportunities or time with friends and family because the restaurant they're going to doesn't offer something that fits in your macros, there's a problem. If you tell your children you won't share an ice cream cone with them because you weren't happy with the number on the scale that day, there's a problem. If you are ignoring your hunger because you have already eaten your allotted calories, macros, or containers for the day, there's a problem.

Why We Cannot Trust Body Weight Scales

I have no idea what I weigh. That's a lie. I have a general idea of the range that I know to be my weight set range. I don't weigh myself, though. I used to be ruled by the scale, and now I don't even keep one in our bathroom. My husband insists on having one in the house for himself, but I don't step on it because I now know it tells me nothing useful about my body or myself.

First, there are so many factors that can affect your weight on any given day. Did you have a lot of salt or carbohydrates the day before? Those will make you retain water. Did you hydrate enough the day before? Have you eliminated all the waste in your body? When was the last time you ate? Are you menstruating? Are you sick? Have you had anything to eat or drink that day? Did you already work out? Are you wearing clothes?

Scales aren't super accurate either. We had two scales in our house at one point and both of them read different numbers. So the version of me who would let a half-pound difference dictate her mood for the day based on that number would be super confused on what to believe and how to feel.

Lastly, what information does the scale actually tell you? Your weight is not tied to your worth. You are not more worthy if you weigh less or are thin and less worthy if you weigh more or live in a larger body. I am probably heavier than I was during and even before my eating disorder. I'm older and I've had a baby, which partially contributes to that fact. But guess what? I love and respect my body more now than I ever did then. If you would've told me then that I would be happy now at this weight, I wouldn't have believed you. But it's true. This work is real and transformative.

What We Can Trust: Our Bodies, with Interoceptive Awareness

Getting to the point I am now with my body and weight may sound impossible to you. The idea of trusting your body sounds laughable.

You've got to this point in your life, frustrated with your body, and even the most restrictive of diets and intense exercise don't lead to the body you want. If you did *quit diets* and *trust your body*, you think you'd be in even worse shape than you believe yourself to be now. Your body clearly cannot be trusted, right?

It's understandable that you would feel that way. Diet culture tells you that their way *is* the only way, and it's your shortcomings to blame for why their way hasn't worked for you. Remember from earlier chapters of this book, though, that studies show diets do not work long-term. Also remember from earlier chapters that diet companies are much more interested in profit than your best interest. Who should you really trust in terms of who has your best interest in mind? You.

Interoceptive awareness is the ability to read, understand, and respond to the body's natural cues. Your body tells you when it needs to cough, sneeze, and urinate; in the same way, it tells you when you're hungry and full. You are more attuned to when you need to pee because you don't try to manipulate that function of your body with shame. You have to go, you go. You don't hold it in telling yourself that you just went an hour ago. You just go. The signal to urinate is very clear to us and we don't second-guess what we need to do to get rid of that signal.

Eating should be the same. When we are hungry, we should be able to read those signals and act accordingly, as it is when we are full and know when to stop. Given our culture, this seems to be decidedly more difficult, so there are ways to increase your interoceptive awareness.

One way to measure your ability for interoceptive awareness is to perceive your heart beating. First, try measuring your pulse by putting two fingers on the inside of your wrist and counting the beats for one minute. Feel the blood pump through your artery. The next step is sitting or lying still and seeing if you can feel your heartbeat in your chest without touching your chest with your hand. This may take some practice to feel without putting your hand there.

Meditation is also a very effective way to build your relationship to your body's cues, and it's a double whammy because it's also a form of self-care that can be super effective in calming the nervous system and slowing down our thoughts. Try a body scan meditation. This is when you inhale and you concentrate on one part of your body, envisioning the air filling up that part of your body; and on the exhale, you completely relax that body part, letting it melt down toward the floor, chair, or bed. Systematically, you move from the top of your head to your toes. In this way, you pay attention to each part of your body and what those parts may need or if you are holding tension in them.

Labeling your body sensations as positive, negative, and neutral can also help develop interoceptive awareness. This labeling can be used in tandem with the hunger—fullness scale, where 0 is ravenously hungry and 10 is uncomfortably full and sick. When you are at a 4, is this positive, negative, or neutral? For me, this is a pleasant feeling of hunger. I am ready to eat. When I'm at a 2, I find this to be a negative feeling, as I am now over hungry; on the other hand, a 9 feels negative in terms of fullness.

Interoceptive awareness takes time. Do not beat yourself up if you are not perfectly in tune with your body and undereat or overeat. You are simply taking steps to learn more about your body. I suggest keeping a diary or a journal for a while to keep track of what happened when you reached different points on the scale, how you felt, what you did as a result, and how that result made you feel. When you reached a 4, did you eat until a 7, and was that experience positive? Did you wait until a 2 and then eat until an 8, and was that experience negative?

If you are someone who no longer has hunger and fullness cues, you can practice feeling both of them using water. Fill up several cups of water, wait until you believe you're hungry—at least neutral—and start slowly drinking the water. Try to tune in to the difference in your stomach as you drink each glass. Notice any feelings of heaviness, pressure, fullness, or tightness.

It's also worth noting here that hunger feels differently for different people. I almost never experience a growling stomach as a hunger signal. Instead, you may feel tired and lethargic, zapped of energy, a dull, gnawing feeling in your stomach, a headache, brain fog, or anxiousness and irritability. It's important to pay attention to those and also to when they occur. Perhaps lightheadedness is your early warning sign of hunger at a 4, which leads to irritability at a 3, and a hunger headache at a 2.

Feeling your fullness before it becomes uncomfortable can be tricky at first, as it takes about twenty minutes for your brain to receive the signal that it is full and satiated. As a result, it's best to eat without distraction. Utilize all five senses when eating to really make it a pleasurable, immersive experience. Many have issues doing this at first because of the shame associated with eating. Try to remind yourself that you are learning how to listen to your body, and that slowing down and learning this skill of interoceptive awareness will actually, with time, decrease your instances of food shame overall. Take a few deep, expansive breaths before you begin eating. Calming the body down before you eat helps calm the parasympathetic system, your "fight or flight" response. Doing this will help your body with digestion and decrease instances of bloating and gas, both of which only increase food shame after eating. Halfway through the meal, pause and put your utensils down. How does your body feel? Is it physically full? Are you mentally satiated? Will another bite serve to end the meal? This is where we look for the "last bite threshold."

A Note for Those With Medical Conditions

You can absolutely be an intuitive eater! The whole point of intuitive eating is feeling good in your body while honoring our mind—body—spirit health. If you have diabetes, for example, you work to manage your blood sugar levels, which would require being mindful of the numbers on your blood glucose meter or a continuous glucose monitor. This is a situation where reading numbers is crucial, not disordered. The intention is very different. Eating "perfectly" won't get you the "perfect" blood sugars, and there is no definitive "diabetes diet." Instead, pay attention to and get curious about how your body feels after you eat certain foods. In fact, a 2021 observational study showed that intuitive eating is associated with glycemic control for those with type 2 diabetes. [26] The same goes for women suffering, for example, from polycystic ovary syndrome (PCOS). Many doctors will prescribe weight loss, but PCOS occurs in normal and underweight women, as well. Moreover, dieting can actually worsen symptoms of PCOS in the long term. Hunger and low blood sugar contribute to anxiety, depression, and fatigue, and those things occur often when following a restrictive diet. Forget low-fat diets with PCOS, too: your body needs adequate dietary fat to create hormones and adequate calories to promote menstruation and fertility. Instead of focusing on an external prescription of rules and regulations, pay attention to how your body feels after you eat certain foods. Your body will tell you exactly what it needs and doesn't need.

---

26. Fabíola Lacerda Pires Soares, Mariana Herzog Ramos, Mariana Gramelisch, Rhaviny de Paula Pego Silva, Jussara da Silva Batista, Monica Cattafesta, and Luciane Bresciani Salaroli, "Intuitive Eating Is Associated with Glycemic Control in Type 2 Diabetes," *Eating and Weight Disorders* 26, no. 2 (March 2021): 599–608, https://doi.org/10.1007/s40519-020-00894-8.

CHAPTER 4:

The Shadow Sides
of Health Pursuits

Most cultures have become hyper-focused on health. You constantly hear about the new superfoods for memory, longevity, sleep, and anything else to improve the things that fall apart thanks to today's go-go-go culture. You should be eating "healthy" and working out, and if you're not actively pursuing these things, you're lazy and irresponsible.

Since the media and those around you are in constant pursuit of better health, you are peer pressured to drink the low-calorie, no sugar Kool-Aid and jump on the health and wellness bandwagon. It's a point of "commissary camaraderie," a point of connection between you and others, a way to bond with the people around you. You feel less miserable about your body, or at least not alone in your misery, when your girlfriends are also complaining about their bodies. And, if they are complaining about their bodies, and you think they have better bodies than you, you begin to wonder if you should feel dissatisfied with yours, too, if you're not already. In 2011, one small study of female college students found that a staggering ninety-three percent of college-age women participate in this type of talk, regardless of their size. [27]

The obsession with longevity adds to perpetuate this quest for optimal health. People want to live forever; the idea of simply not existing rightfully scares them into doing anything and everything that will extend their lives. And what's more, they want to live longer without pain or illness holding them back.

So, how has the idea of health and longevity translated into an aesthetic, an image? Through diet culture's constant messaging of what they believe to be health, an "ideal picture of health" has been created. It's thin, it's young-looking, it's active, it's happy. So, to be healthy has become synonymous with being all of these other things, as well, so much so that being young-looking and thin has actually *replaced* true health and longevity.

A huge breakthrough in my food freedom journey was realizing that being thin and being healthy can be, and many times are, mutually exclusive; especially if the thinness is unnatural to one's particular body type and genetics.

When I was a disordered eater, I was, according to the BMI scale, still a relatively "normal" weight; however, the better indicator that this wasn't an appropriate weight for me was how hard I had to struggle and starve myself to stay there. I exhibited very disordered and disturbing behaviors to maintain that weight. I had troubling and obsessive thoughts while maintaining that weight. Looking back on it, I was the opposite of the picture of health.

My physical health was deteriorating as a result of trying to achieve a certain weight and six-pack abs. My fingernails were brittle and had these deep, horizontal ridges in them; it turns out the structure of

---

27. Aubrey Gordon, "It's Time for a Culture of Consent Around Body Talk," *SELF*, August 27, 2020, http://www.self.com/story/body-talk-consent.

human nails are altered with malnutrition. They looked like little washboards. I remember Googling why my nails looked all weird all of a sudden, and I recall blowing off the idea that it could be a symptom of malnourishment. How could I be malnourished when I ate healthy foods? Of course, I was in denial that I wasn't eating *enough* food at all.

Even more baffling to me was my elevated LDL cholesterol, commonly referred to as "bad" cholesterol. When I spoke to my general practitioner about my concerns, he shrugged and said, "Well, the rest of your blood work looks okay. You don't smoke, so just continue to eat healthy and exercise." Talk about triggering. Was I not eating healthy *enough?* Was I not exercising *enough?*

I had brain fog all the time; even the mental math needed to calculate my daily calories was difficult. Concentrating on anything for sustained periods of time was exhausting. On top of that, the constant thoughts around food blocked any other thoughts from being processed. While out to lunch with a friend, she would be gushing about her new boyfriend and how happy he made her—and all I could think about was how happy the "cheat" food I had ordered was about to make me. Or I was secretly regretting the fact that I ordered a "safe" option when I really wanted the "cheat" option. Or I was doing mental math to reassure myself that this meal wasn't going to derail my goals.

Lethargy from insufficient caloric intake made me feel as if my whole day was trudging through wet cement. I remember the walk up the two flights of stairs to my tiny, attic apartment was difficult, which struck me as odd, considering I worked out at the gym every day. I always felt lightheaded by the time I reached the top.

Aside from physical issues, my mental health, ironically, was suffering in my quest for "optimal health." I weighed myself obsessively, every morning. I looked forward to the weigh-in, praying for a lower number than the day before. I had to do it first thing in the morning, fully naked, before I had even a sip of water. I remember days where I'd weigh myself, and have to reweigh myself because I noticed my hair tie was still on my wrist the first time. Most anxiety-inducing in creating the perfect environment for a weigh-in, though, was whether I had a bowel movement. If I actually didn't have to go, I would sit there and strain to produce one or use an enema.

This weigh-in dictated the tone for the rest of my day. If I was lighter than the day before, I was elated and moved into the rest of my day with a sick sense of accomplishment. I was on the path to "success" and gave myself the proverbial gold star.

If I was heavier than the day before, especially if it was more than a pound, all hell would break loose in my head. Where did I go wrong? What do I need to do today to fix this? What do I need to cut out of my diet today to make up for this, or how much longer should I run on the treadmill? If I had plans to go to lunch or dinner with a friend, I suddenly wondered if I should cancel, because eating out would surely only make things worse the following morning.

I wouldn't allow myself to make plans on back-to-back days with friends or my partner either. That was too many cheat meals in one week. And forget any semblance of spontaneity. I would never go out for drinks with coworkers after work because those drinks didn't fit into my calorie count for the day, or if they did, I'd have to skip my afternoon snack and would never make it to dinner without binge eating whatever appetizers my coworkers ordered.

I would obsessively think about food, whether it was what I just ate, what I was eating, or what I would eat at my next meal. Food was my past, present, and future. There wasn't room to think about anything else.

It's not even surprising, really. The famous Minnesota Starvation study saw 36 men voluntarily starve themselves by cutting their caloric intake in half, to roughly 1,600 a day. The study showed that the men became obsessed with food. "During the semi-starvation phase, the changes were dramatic. Beyond the gaunt appearance of the men, there were significant decreases in their strength and stamina, body temperature, heart rate, and sex drive. The psychological effects were significant as well. Hunger made the men obsessed with food. They would dream and fantasize about food, read and talk about food and savor the two meals a day they were given. They reported fatigue, irritability, depression, and apathy."[28]

I know what you're thinking: "My diet/coach/calorie calculator tells me to eat 1,600 a day for my body size!" ... exactly. Yes, men typically require more calories than women, but the difference in caloric needs between genders is not vast enough that what is considered starvation for one can be considered appropriate for the other. This study proves that the diet industry is trying to starve us out, keep us preoccupied with our bodies and their programs, and make our brains fuzzy so we can't think about how absolutely bananas all of this is. They won't even *allow* bananas!

Now, weight loss may be a good thing *if you're above your weight set range;* and no, that's not the range an online calculator tells you. Perhaps you've been binge eating and that's caused weight gain. Maybe you use food often to numb out or soothe unpleasant emotions, and that's caused weight gain. In these cases, weight loss is a good thing, not as a primary goal but as a byproduct of healing inner wounds; but clearly, as I've seen through personal experience, there can be too much of a "good thing." If you're approaching weight loss as an active goal, you are typically doing so because you have attached self-worth to your aesthetic; and in that case, as

---

28. David B. Baker and Natacha Keramidas, "The Psychology of Hunger," *Monitor on Psychology 44, no. 9 (October 2013):* 66, http://www.apa.org/monitor/2013/10/hunger.

it was in mine, no amount of weight loss will fix that desire for self-worth.

Eating whole, unprocessed foods is a good thing, if you are someone who can financially afford it. From a nutritional profile perspective, whole, unprocessed foods are the better choice *most of the time*. Organic foods are the better choice *most of the time*; but if we are micromanaging every bite that goes into our mouths and having legitimate fears around foods that are not up to our impossibly high standards of consumption, is that still a good thing? I would wager it's not. Also, when I say these are the better choices, I do not mean to assign morality to them. Keep in mind that organic foods still have pesticides on them, and some processed foods like protein powders can be nutrient-dense. When the desire for something like organic, unprocessed, non-GMO foods becomes obsessive and rigid, it is no longer a healthy practice. In fact, there's a different name for it: orthorexia. Orthorexia is defined as an unhealthy obsession with healthy eating, and trust me when I say, there are few boxes smaller than the one you put yourself in when you become orthorexic.

The life I was living with orthorexia was horrible and disordered. This was not the way life was meant to be lived. If your mental sanity is the price you pay in the pursuit of achieving a certain body size or shape, is it even worth it anymore? Can you even enjoy it? If the answer for you is still yes, I would reread Chapter 2 and then read on to the chapter after this one to figure out your true why, and do some thought work to heal the things that are ailing your soul. You won't find the answers in a different body. This is why we see thin, beautiful people who are still tragically self-loathing; conversely, this is why we also see some people in larger bodies being the most confident, self-assured people in the room. Thinness doesn't equal happiness or confidence.

When I was in grad school, I was on this quest for peak health. To pay for school, I had a graduate assistantship in the English department of my college. When there was a lull in the work to be done, I would scour the Internet for articles about health and how to optimize it: have better skin, gain more muscle, lose weight, burn fat, increase longevity, improve memory ... basically be a robot human. I was obsessed with following the advice in these articles, which typically came from popular "health and wellness" websites or magazines and not scientific studies.

Having knowledge of true health, fitness, and nutrition can be a wonderful thing, as opposed to the bastardized versions that diet culture glorifies. As a teacher, I am a "forever learner" and encourage others to do the same. But this hyperfocus I had on health and obsession with reading health articles was indicative of a preoccupation with my weight and body and a disordered goal of perfection. It's one thing to occasionally read an interesting article; it's quite another to scour the Internet for hours.

This "more is better" attitude can also stem from, or even create, perfectionism and obsessive-compulsive disorder (OCD). You become so rigid in your thinking and behaviors that you will punish yourself for any time you spill out of the very small box you've stuffed yourself in; and you will, usually in the form of binge eating.

If my story and past behaviors resonate with you, there are three key ways to break these binge—restrict cycles. If you're experiencing orthorexia, there's a really good chance you're experiencing binge—restrict cycles. I know this was my experience, and I know other women, as well, who have been through the same thing. When you are white-knuckling through your weeks eating nothing but raw vegetables and hard boiled eggs, by week's end, you are craving pizza, cheese, pasta ... whatever your go-to "cheat" meal is. You swear you're only going to have an "appropriate" amount, but that never happens. When you're in a binge state, it feels like your brain has been hijacked, and you can't stop yourself. You can't even think straight to stop yourself. When you finally come up for air, you feel uncomfortably full, out of control, frustrated, shameful, and fearful of "undoing" your progress. The best case scenario is you tell yourself that tomorrow you will be "better," only to perpetuate the binge—restrict cycle again. Worst case scenario, you turn to eating disorder behaviors like purging.

If you're suffering with binge eating, here are four steps to breaking the cycle.

Breaking the Binge Cycle Step #1: Stop Restricting

Unfortunately, the only true antidote for breaking the binge—restrict cycle is to stop restricting. I say "unfortunately" because I know this goes against what you instinctively want to do after a binge; you want to balance out the scales. All this will do, though, is set you up for the next binge.

But what about willpower? I just need strong willpower, right?

Diet culture leads you to believe that diets, especially restrictive ones, fail because *you* failed. You were the problem. You weren't strong enough or determined enough to make it work. That's a bald-faced lie. Binge eating after restriction is a biological response to starvation. Again, the body doesn't know the difference between famine and a diet. Fighting a binge is like fighting the urge to urinate ... eventually your body is just going to do what it needs to do to survive, whether you want it to or not.

So the only way to stop the cycle is by doing something brave and different: Don't restrict.

Breaking the Binge Cycle Step #2:
Stop Counting Calories and Macros

You'll want to restrict if you pay attention to calorie or macro counts. You're going to get anxious and want to start planning the rest of your day around how many calories are left. You're going to try to land in that calorie deficit to lose weight. You're going to start using your head and its disordered calculations instead of your heart and your stomach to guide your food choices. Relying on calorie or macro counts, or any external tool, is a restriction against what your body needs. Instead, try to use the hunger-fullness scale, a 0–10 scale intuitive eaters use to assess their hunger and fullness. Using this scale can be difficult for those who have been chronically restricting and no longer accurately feel hunger and fullness cues. In order to regain those sensations, aim to nourish your body every three to four hours, even if you don't feel hunger. When you are eating, eliminate distractions around you to be mindful of your experience. Eat slowly and stop halfway through to check on your fullness and satiety level. Once your metabolism has been reset through this process of eating consistently, you can begin to determine what levels of hunger and fullness feel pleasant for you. For me, I like to eat around 3–4 and stop around 7.

Breaking the Binge Cycle Step #3:
Listen to Your Body's Cues

Are you hungry? If the answer is yes, eat. What are you hungry for? Notice I didn't ask, "What *should* you eat?" There are no "shoulds" in intuitive eating. How will you feel *in your body* after you eat it? Again, I didn't say, "How will your mind feel?" If you are early in recovery, chances are we already know that if you honor your cravings, you will feel anxious, scared, and guilty. But we want to get you out of your head and into your body. The thoughts you experience when you are honoring your cravings in the beginning should be journaled. Apply the why game to them and always be conscious of where your thoughts are coming from.

Breaking the Binge Cycle Step #4: Rewire Thoughts with Repetition

The only reason you should still be in your head is to keep repeating affirmations that will help you along in this process. *Restriction got me here; it won't get me out.* When you want to restrict, remind yourself repeatedly that restriction is the reason you keep binge eating in the first place; it's worth noting here, as well, that past trauma and a lack of coping mechanisms are additional common reasons people can experience BED. *Consistent nourishment gives me energy and mental clarity.* Repeat to yourself the benefits of consistent meals.

I advise against toxic positivity when it comes to repetition and affirmations. If you're in a place where you hate your body, repeating, "I love my body" on loop won't be effective. It will feel inauthentic and will actually do more harm than good when you realize you wholeheartedly disagree with that thought. Instead, think of body thoughts on a spectrum from self-hate to self-love. In between those two ends are neutrality and self-acceptance. Try on different phrases and affirmations until you find ones that are one step closer to self-love but also genuinely resonate with you. Some examples might be, "I have a body," "I appreciate what my body can do," or "All humans have different bodies."

CHAPTER 5:

Creating Your Nutrition Goals
as an Intuitive Eater

We live in such a fast-paced culture. We work the majority of our days, with many of us working more than one job. We take care of children or other loved ones; and yes, pets definitely count. And at the end of the day, we still attempt to carve out time that is just ours, whether we use that to exercise, sleep, or binge-watch Netflix.

It's no wonder most of us have no clue what our "why" is when it comes to nutrition and fitness. We don't even have time to stop and reflect on it!

If you have a disordered relationship with food and fitness, you probably haven't thought very much past the fact you want to have a flat stomach and to meet some arbitrary goal weight. And those should be enough, right? Those are what you want, and therefore, you count calories, eat clean, and work out so you can have those things, right?

If you've been even remotely conscious for the first few chapters of this book, you now know that these superficial reasons for wanting to diet are not the real reasons. Even your relationship with fitness has never really been about the actual size and shape of your body. More often than not, disordered behaviors around food and movement are created because of messages we're told by society. Those messages, heard over and over, become internalized as part of our narrative and our perceived truth. We're told our body's size and shape are a problem to be solved, and diet companies are selling the solutions to those problems.

When I was in my twenties, I wanted to be as thin as possible, so I ate as little as possible. That was seriously my goal, and that was seriously as deep as I thought about it. Eventually, I replaced that goal with the goal to "get healthy," so I ate more food, but *only* "clean" food. "Getting healthy" and "eating clean" sound like noble goals, right?

When your goal is to eat clean *all* the time, the restriction you experience will not only damage your body when you inevitably binge, but it will also damage your mental health and erode the trust between your mind and your body. By the weekend, I was mentally and physically exhausted, so I naturally would binge on the macronutrient that gives people the most energy: carbs. Chips, pretzels, ice cream, you name it. This was usually after having a cocktail or two so my inhibitions were lowered, and I felt I could allow myself the binge; heck, I deserved it after being so "good" all week! The weekend binges I experienced were a natural bodily response, given they typically followed a week of eating nothing but oatmeal, egg whites, almond butter, chicken, and vegetables.

My "why" was vague, it was underdeveloped, it was disordered, and it wasn't even the core why! My "why" during the thick of my eating disorder was to weigh as little as possible. Not only was this a reason that wasn't rooted in love or respect for myself, it also didn't make logical sense. It had no end, and if I kept trying to pursue it, I would eventually end up in a treatment center or dead. What I was really chasing with that why was the external validation that I was beautiful, and by extension, worthy.

My "why" now with food, body, and fitness looks much different and is no longer black and white. It is one that embraces "and." I want to be physically strong using exercise, *and* I want fitness to be only one part of my day. I want to live a long life, *and* I want to have fun while doing it. I want to show my son, Archer, what a strong woman looks like: body, mind, *and* spirit. I want to eat foods that nourish my body *and* enjoy foods that satiate me.

So, here are the four steps you can follow to figure out the *true* reason behind your disordered eating.

Why Game Step #1: Define Your Goal

What is your goal? Is it to lose fifteen pounds? Is it to fit into a size six dress? Is it to feel sexy? Whatever it is, know that there is no judgment with this initial goal. You may just be starting this work for the first time, and I want to meet you where you're at. I totally understand why your goal is your goal, and it's only natural when society has told you that it *should* be your goal! So, without fear or shame, write that bad boy down.

Why Game Step #2: Ask Yourself Why That's Your Goal

You may have even considered a step past Step 1! You just figured, "I want to lose fifteen pounds," and didn't think much about that goal because, hey, basically all your friends are looking to be skinnier, too. But seriously, why *are* you looking to lose those fifteen pounds? Typically, the answer is something like, "Because that's what I was in college," or "I'm currently overweight." You know your truth, so be honest about it.

Why Game Step #3: Ask Yourself Why AGAIN

At the risk of sounding repetitive or facetious, I want you to ask yourself "why" again. If the answer to Step 2 was, "Because that's the size/weight I was in college," ask yourself, "*Why* do I need to be the same size/weight that I was in college?" Is it because you're looking to have your youth, or rather, society's version of youth, back? Is it because it was a freer, simpler time for you? Were you validated in college with good grades or athletic accomplishments and want to feel special again? Again, this type of deep thought work may dig up some feelings of shame when you realize where your goals are really coming from. Resist the urge to go down a shame spiral. Society has conditioned you to have these deeper reasons for wanting weight loss so the fact you even want to unlearn this condition puts you ahead of the curve, trust me.

If the answer was, "I'm overweight," ask yourself, "Well, why is it bad to be overweight?" Over *what* weight, and by whose standards? Do you feel bad physically in your "overweight" body, or do you feel bad because people in your life or your potentially fatphobic doctor have told you that you *should* feel bad? In Chapter 2, we saw how Body Mass Index (BMI) is an inaccurate measure of what someone "should" weigh and why it should not be a standard barometer of health.

Why Game Step #4: Ask Yourself, "What Is Another Way I Can Fulfill This Need for SALV (Safety, Acceptance, Love, Validation) that's Not Related to My Weight or Body?"

No doubt we all seek safety, acceptance, love, and validation, or as I like to call it, SALV, like the salve you apply to a wound. I sure do, and I would never deny anyone from desiring or seeking out those things. We're human, after all; but is there any other way you can fulfill SALV without fixating on your weight or body? For example, I'm someone who has been conditioned to seek validation through her looks since I was a child; now, I try to focus more on being validated through my roles as a mom and teacher. I've also tried to focus on cultivating more internal validation, reminding myself that we are all born with inherent value, and that my failures do not take away from that value; and mindset is everything. In fact, I can choose to see my failures as a testament to my courage to fail and determination to meet my goals. If I want to feel sexy, I'll put on an outfit that's comfortable and I feel confident in. If I want to feel loved, I hang out with my husband or my son. If I want to feel heard, I can write a post on social media for my followers or in my gratitude journal. There are so many ways to go about finding things that will uniquely "fill your cup" that are not related to aesthetic validation.

Beware Disordered Nutrition Goals

You don't want nutrition goals to be about aesthetics. You don't want them to be about looking thin, or having a flat stomach, or a thigh gap. The reason you don't want these to be your goals is because they focus on your external value and only cultivate temporary external validation in a society that applauds these things; they are not a measure of health either, so don't try to use the "I'm just trying to be healthy" cop-out to justify your current aesthetic goals. We also don't want to focus on external gains because those can be taken away. Suppose tomorrow you are in a horrible accident that leaves you paralyzed from the neck down. No more exercise. No more hopes of a conventionally perfect body. Will your value and self-worth crumble in the face of losing your only, or your biggest, mode of validation?

With that scenario in mind, when considering your nutrition goals, focus on how your body *feels*. When I stopped calorie counting and started honoring my hunger and fullness, I could not believe the shift in my energy levels. I felt refreshed and alive, as if someone had opened the door and a rush of cool air hit my face. The brain fog lifted, and I didn't feel like I was spending my entire day walking through quick-sand anymore. An effective question to ask yourself if you're afraid your goal may be disordered is: Does this goal seek to make me *feel* good in my body? Or does this goal seek to only make me *look* good in my body? The latter, as you may have guessed, is the disordered one.

Why Eating Disorder Recovery Is So Difficult ... and a Focus on Intention

This can be terrifyingly hard work, especially because eating disorders are unique from any other disorder that revolves around obsession. Unlike alcoholism or drug addiction, the "substance" in question—food—is unavoidable. Alcohol and drugs are not necessary for surviv-al, but food is, and you have to face it several times a day, every single day.

Creating nutritional goals in the name of authentic health needs to first be done from a healthy *mindset*. Although I created "nutritional goals" during my ED, they clearly were not being created with a healthy *mindset*. They were being created by a voice inside me telling me I wasn't perfect enough yet, and therefore, not yet worthy.

After reading this book, you may change your why for nutrition and fitness, but some behaviors may stay the same. That is *not* an in-vitation to continue eating 1,200 calories. Some behaviors, no matter how you cut it, are disordered.

Two people can eat the same amount of food, even the *same* foods, and their intentions can completely color whether they're approaching their nutrition from a place of self-love or self-hate. If someone eats a big piece of cake at a birthday party, they might be doing so because the idea of cake sounds delicious to them at the moment; they know their body will feel okay afterward, and they are not placing value on the cake as "healthy" or "unhealthy." Someone else, on the other hand, might be having a big piece of cake because they already feel like they "cheated" with the dinner they also just enjoyed; since they were already "bad," they might as well continue to be bad and start over tomorrow. The cake is not enjoyed but used as a mode of self-punishing, self-fulfilling prophecy.

Intention is everything; and it is something you should revisit often. Are you still doing the things in your day-to-day life for the right reasons?

The Roles of Food and Grace in Our Lives

You also have to remember that food is not just to live. If you're hyper-focused on an aesthetic goal or weight, you may believe things like, "Well, food is just for survival, so that's how I'm going to treat it in order to meet my aesthetic goals," "I now eat to live," or, "Food is just fuel."

Hard pass. Food is one of the most exciting and special parts of life! It brings us together with family and friends. It's used to celebrate milestones, create new memories, bond with others, pass down traditions, and color our varied cultures.

To strip down food to a mere requirement for survival hinders its ability to foster happiness, memories, and relationships; you don't want to attend social events anymore because they become anxiety-inducing, threatening to sabotage your body goals. If you agree to go, you find it difficult to be present-minded, preoccupied with white-knuckling your "willpower" to not "cheat" on your diet; but each time you turn down plans to go out, you turn more inward to your own thoughts, including the disordered ones, away from those who love you, and away from human connection; this isolation is where shame loves to breed.

Diet culture can also make you feel such shame for not seeing eating as strictly utilitarian. It's totally okay to use food for moral support or comfort sometimes! Again, you're a grown adult with the ability to make your own decisions. However, I do recommend that you be intentional and mindful about it. You are allowed to feel whatever emotion you want or need to feel, and once you've intentionally processed that emotion, you can intentionally engage in whatever feels like self-care in the moment, including eating ice cream.

Sugar only feels addictive because it lights up what's called the mesolimbic dopamine system. Dopamine is a brain chemical released by neurons that tells the brain that you've had a positive experience, like eating sugar.[29] In very rare cases are people actually addicted to sugar; instead it simply feels that way because we've been conditioned to fear and restrict it. After the occasional rough day at work, I've intentionally eaten chocolate or chips to make myself feel better; "intentionally" being the operative word. I first acknowledge whatever emotion I'm feeling, whether it's frustration or anxiety, etc., and then I intentionally decide that chocolate will be my coping mechanism that day, just one of the many that I have in my "toolbox." I'll mindfully eat the chocolate, stay in touch with how my body feels as I eat it, savor it, and move on.

As I've said before, this work is tough and nuanced. You are working against the current wiring of your brain, which is constantly flooded

---

29. Amy Reichelt, "Your Brain on Sugar: What the Science Actually Says," *The Conversation*, November 14, 2019, https://theconversation.com/your-brain-on-sugar-what-the-science-actually-says-126581.

with messages from social media, culture, friends, and family. There's only a small community of us who know the truth: that diet culture is toxic and was never the antidote to the issues you are experiencing with self-acceptance.

With this in mind, give yourself patience and grace. Take this work one step at a time, one day at a time, one meal at a time, one small win at a time. The journey is not linear. You will backslide. I'm very vocal about this on Instagram. I *still* have one-off days when I can hear the old thoughts creeping in. Do not beat yourself up because we—those who have successfully healed—have all been there. It's whether you get back up that matters, no matter how many times you have to do it. The only way to fail is to stop trying. If you continue to work on this practice, you can't ever truly fail. Accept where you're at, no matter where that is, and take the next step forward toward a future of acceptance, love, and peace.

Examples of Nutrition Goals as an Intuitive Eater

Once you've discovered your reasons and intentions for wanting to adopt a nutrition goal, you can start the work of making one. You don't have to wait to heal the issues that are creating a disordered relationship with food and your body to create a nutrition goal; in fact, setting and meeting non-diet nutrition goals can be super empowering in terms of showing you how great you can feel in your body when you're not chasing weight loss.

Although perhaps obvious at this point, I recommend approaching nutrition goals from a place of abundance and not scarcity. Your goal shouldn't be to cut or restrict any food or food group. If numbers are triggering to you, I also suggest keeping them out of your goals. Instead of taking things out as a form of punishment, focus on adding things in as a form of self-care. Maybe your goal is to try one new fruit or vegetable every two weeks. Try a new recipe every week. Drink more water consistently throughout the day. Add more vegetables that you love. Aim to eat every 3–4 hours. Aim to create meals that include all three macronutrients: carbohydrates, fats, and protein. Those are goals that truly nourish and take care of your body instead of punishing it and limiting it.

You may have noticed that although this chapter was titled "Creating Your Nutrition Goals as an Intuitive Eater," I only got to actual intuitive eating nutrition goals in the last page; this is intentional. The most difficult and time-consuming part of being an intuitive eater is wading through and challenging all the muck that diet culture has thrown in front of you. Once you can see past all of that, intuitive eating becomes fascinatingly simple.

CHAPTER 6

Practical Tips for Transitioning to Food Freedom

Having all this freedom with food, as a new intuitive eater, can be overwhelming. There are a lot of fear foods to reintroduce and food rules, like not eating after 7 p.m., to throw out the window; here are fifteen tricks to making the transition from diet land a little smoother.

Transition Tip #1: Only Eat It if You Really Want It, Not because It's There or You Feel You're Not Eating Intuitively by Not Having It.

If you restrict your food or certain food groups, you may experience "last supper mentality." Last supper mentality is when you feel this uncontrollable need to finish whatever food is in front of you because you've decided it's the last time you can have it. For example, you could be having a nice dinner out with your partner and feel the need to finish everything on your plate because you don't allow yourself to eat that kind of food when you're at home. You're full, but it tastes so good, and you know this is your only chance to enjoy it. You might also have occasions where food left on your plate that's not quite enough for a leftover meal but you would feel guilty throwing it out. This type of behavior is common with people who experience food insecurity as children or any other forms of food scarcity. Or you might eat a slice of cake for a colleague's birthday, even though it doesn't really taste good or isn't a flavor you enjoy, but you've saved up calories ahead of time for this "cheat."

No matter the reason, the last supper mentality needs to be quieted in order to truly experience intuitive eating and food freedom. Eating intuitively is about what you want to eat and how you feel when you eat it, not eating what you feel obligated to eat. Like anything else, navigating this new terrain takes practice and grace ... and a few tips!

First, ask yourself: *Is this really something I want?* If the answer is *yes*, have it! Intuitive eaters honor all hunger, including taste hunger, which is eating just because it sounds yummy! The next question to ask is, *Do I want it only because the opportunity presented itself but I actually don't like it?* If the answer is *yes*, don't have it. I fell into this a lot in the beginning of my intuitive eating journey. My coworker friend once baked a chocolate cake at home and left a piece in my mailbox at work because she knows I have a sweet tooth. The thing is, she didn't know I don't like chocolate cake. I know, I know, how am I even human? I love chocolate, just not chocolate cake. Back in the day, I would eat it just because it was something I normally wouldn't allow myself anywhere near. Now, I take a bite just so I can have something specific and complimentary to say about it when I thank her, and then, I throw the rest out. If it was something larger, like an entire chocolate cake made for me, instead of throwing it out, I would put it in the faculty room for others to enjoy.

I am not afraid of the chocolate cake, fearful of the calories, or anxious how "unhealthy" it is. It's just that I know I typically don't like chocolate cake. Don't get me wrong; if I had taken a bite and thought it was delicious, I would've saved it for later, after dinner, with a hot cup of tea. But I'm not going to eat something I don't truly enjoy just because it was given to me or because I am an intuitive eater. That's something many rookie intuitive eaters do; they feel this pressure to eat the "junk" foods because now they have given themselves permission to, and they're afraid that if they don't eat those foods, they're still restricting. Not so. Again, it's all about intention: if you're choosing foods based on hunger and preference, not fear of weight gain, you can choose whatever makes you happy!

Transition Tip #2: If You're Eating Out, Portion Some of Your Dinner on a Smaller Plate; and if You Want More After That, Go for It!

A huge part of conquering binge eating is to make sure all foods are available, all the time. Let's say you go out to dinner at a fancy restaurant; you might not be able to get their world-famous risotto every time you want it because it's expensive, and you can't always get the babysitter to watch the kids. I get it. But you also don't want to binge on it because then you'll feel guilty and feel the urge to restrict afterward.

When I first started intuitively eating, I would ask the wait staff for a smaller plate. Typically, I know that eating an entire restaurant portion of food will make me uncomfortably full. I also know that eating with company can result in mindless, distracted eating. So I put what I *think* will make me full and satiated onto the smaller plate. I've become very in tune with my body's typical needs, so it's easy for me to make an educated guess. I eat slowly and mindfully but throw most of my attention into the conversation with my company. When I finish what's on the small plate, I wait a few minutes to check in. Am

I full? Am I satiated? Do I want a few more bites just because it tastes good?

It's okay to say *yes* to that last question, by the way. If I'm still hungry, I honor that physical and/or taste hunger, as long as I don't think it'll leave me uncomfortably full. And that's the key. You can use what diet culture coined "portion control," as long as you don't feel obligated to only eat that amount and know you can have more. It's just a "starting-off point."

Transition Tip #3: Order and Eat What You Want, but Pair It with a Beloved, Nutrient-Dense Food

Let's go back to the risotto example. Who doesn't like a nice, heaping plate of warm risotto? Let's be honest, though; it's not the most nutrient-dense item on the menu. And that's totally fine! You're allowed to have the risotto! But if you know a whole plate of risotto is going to cause intestinal issues or sit heavily in your stomach, pair it with a side of your favorite vegetable or a lean protein; trust me, if it's on the menu, they can make a side order of it. When I get risotto, I get it with salmon and mixed vegetables on top. If I can't finish it, it makes a great breakfast or lunch the next day. Another facet of allowing all foods is allowing them any time you want them. This will help ease that last supper mentality; you know you can have that meal as many times as you want it.

Other common ways I utilize this tip are when my husband, Scott, and I order pizza delivery; I'll make a small side salad with chicken on top to go along with my slice(s) of pizza; or when I have a brownie, I'll have a smaller piece and pair it with a Greek vanilla yogurt. By balancing out the macronutrients of my meals, I will feel fuller and more satiated, longer. Now, it doesn't always have to be a side chicken salad or a side Greek yogurt. It could be roasted veggies with pizza, or meatballs with pizza, or whatever! Whatever nutrient-dense food that also *sounds as good to me as pizza* at the moment. And again, if I'm not still full or satiated, I can go back for more pizza or brownies! I can have more and not feel guilty about it, but I like to start by pairing these foods with more nutrient-dense foods because I know my body will feel more energized afterward.

Transition Tip #4: If You're Eating Out, Bring Home the Leftovers

The reason I'm able to walk away from foods I love when I'm out to dinner or at a party is I know that it isn't the only time I can have them. I can eat more later on that night, or the next night or the next, if I have the leftovers wrapped up. You can wrap up basically anything; seriously, if the bread basket is amazing, I'll have the wait staff wrap that up, too. Don't be shy, because it's either in your belly or in a garbage can. Again, it's all about eliminating the feeling that you can never have that food again. It's eliminating the feeling of deprivation and restriction that's going to free you from binge eating.

Transition Tip #5: Conduct Some Food Experiments and Their Impact on Your Energy Levels

Some in the anti-diet space gawk at the idea of eating anything steamed, baked, or grilled that's typically fried. They see these ways of cooking as diet culture tactics. I disagree. Each method of cooking has its place, and everyone has their preferences. I'll say it until I'm blue in the face: If it's a food preference you have because it pleases your taste buds and makes you feel good in your body after eating it, that's totally fine. The same way you don't want to be bullied by those who subscribe to diet culture, you don't want to be bullied by those who are anti-diet either.

I get pushback on social media any time I have egg whites. I love egg white omelets. I also love hard-boiled eggs and whole, scrambled eggs. I love brownies made with butter, sugar, and flour; I also love them made with black beans and applesauce. Don't let either camp tell you you're not allowed to like the foods you enjoy. This is your journey, not theirs.

All of these food anecdotes are simply experiments I've conducted with my eating habits, seeing what foods feel better in my body but still satiate me: the "real thing" or the "swap." If the swap honestly tastes good to me, I'll take that; if I know it'll lead to a binge later or a lack of satiety, I won't. People have come at me on social media regarding using Greek yogurt as a replacement for sour cream. Truth be told, I can take either in terms of taste, but we always have Greek yogurt in the house, so instead of buying sour cream and using only two scoops, I have Greek yogurt readily available all the time because I use it more often for other meals, too.

Here's an example of one of my *failed* experiments: yam noodles, otherwise known as the "zero calorie" noodles. I was obsessed with these during my eating disorder. Would I ever eat them out of sheer pleasure of their taste? No. That's a swap that, now that I eat intuitively, I would never make. I would much rather have regular pasta, thank you very much; although I do also love spaghetti squash! Same goes for cauliflower pizza. I tried so hard to like homemade cauliflower crust, but I'm Italian ... and there's just no way for that crust to break in half the way a good, well done, gluten dough crust can. Again, though, there are certain brands of cauliflower pizza that are delicious.

In the same way, I prefer most meats grilled, blackened, or baked. I think they're juicier baked, and I loved the blackened edges of anything grilled. Those are "healthy" alternatives to deep frying that I genuinely enjoy and don't leave me feeling deprived. Fried foods can leave me with digestive issues for days, so I typically avoid them.

It's all trial and error. View your journey as if you are a food scientist and you're conducting experiments with your body. See what tastes good and what doesn't. See what feels good and what doesn't. Take notes! And don't worry about what others think; they have their own preferences, and any comments they make about your choices, positively or negatively, are probably steeped in their own diet culture or their jealousy over the fact you have freed yourself from that restrictive, rule-based life.

Transition Tip #6: Freeze Leftovers or Fresh Foods for Later

I always seem to have a student each year who has a penchant for baking and uses me as their culinary guinea pig. Twist my arm, why don't you? For the past few years, I've had a student whose specialty is "slutty brownies," which are a concoction of brownie, chocolate chip cookie, and Oreo cookie. On two occasions this year, she's made me a whole tray of them.

This would have sent me into an anxiety spiral back during my eating disorder. I wouldn't have known whether to throw them all out or shove them all in my mouth before my brain could tell me, "No." Since I *love* these brownies, I can't eat one and throw the rest out like with chocolate cake. Instead, I portion out the brownies, wrap them in cellophane, and freeze them. They freeze really well, and in fact, most baked goods that you freeze take on a denser consistency that, I think, makes them taste even better. I found this out when I portioned, froze, and ate my wedding cake every week for an entire year. By doing this, the baked goods last a lot longer, and I don't feel pressure to have them when I don't want them because I know they're always in my freezer. No more last supper mentality! Allowing all food! Heck, sometimes I *forget* that they're even there! That's true food freedom.

There are very few things that can't be frozen. There are so many meals—breakfast, lunch and dinner—that can be frozen and saved for later. This is far and away my favorite strategy for quick meals and saving foods I'm not ready to eat yet.

Desserts aside, I also utilize the freezer often when I know I'm about to enter a busy season. To prepare for the first few weeks after my son was born, I whipped up a bunch of slow cooker meals, portioned out two servings in each freezer-safe bag for Scott and me, and laid them flat to freeze and store. Current and future moms, those meals really help in those first few weeks when you're sleep-deprived and trying to find your new rhythm and schedule. Otherwise, postpartum can spell trouble for a woman's diet. You're learning how to keep this tiny human alive, you haven't slept, and you've barely had time to shower. This creates an environment where you're not practicing proper self-care. You're waiting way too long to eat and then mindlessly grabbing whatever is in front of you. Meal prepping and freezing in anticipation for these busier seasons of our lives is a form of self-care.

I also very often buy meat like chicken breasts and ground turkey and freeze them; typically you're only supposed to leave raw meat in the fridge for one or two days, and sometimes I won't cook the meat until later in the week. I also tend to make baked turkey meatballs in two- or even three-pound batches, portion out two servings per freezer bag, and freeze them for when we want spaghetti and meatballs or power bowls. When a recipe calls for only one cup of chicken broth or one tablespoon of tomato paste, I'll freeze the rest.

Transition Tip #7: If You Spend Most of Your Days Outside of the House, Meal Prep and Use "Bases" that are Easily Customizable on the Fly

Many people ask how meal planning and prepping can align with intuitive eating. How will you know on Sunday what you'll want to eat for breakfast and lunch all week? That's a tough question. Since I eat breakfast, lunch, and a snack at work, it's also a necessary question for me, so here are some ways I'm always guaranteed yummy food on-the-go.

I have a list of tried and true recipes and combinations that I like to eat. If I look at the list and see I haven't made a certain meal in a while, I will add it to the coming week's meal options. I also try to choose meal options that can be customized easily. For example, power bowls are simply a carb, a protein, and a vegetable with sauce. Maybe you want sweet potatoes as your carb base for half the week and rice for the other half. Or broccoli for half and butternut squash for half. Maybe you have two different sauces you can alternate with. Salads work really well with this idea, too. Even breakfasts can be tailored this way. If you like oatmeal, make a batch for each day of the week and when you wake up to get ready for work, have a variety of toppings on hand that you can put onto the oatmeal: dried fruit, nuts, nut butters, coconut, fresh fruit, granola, etc. Same goes for protein shakes. There are different flavored powders you can blend together with different nut butters, frozen fruits, and flavor extracts to make dozens of different delicious combinations.

Anything that saves me time with a full-time job and a toddler is golden in my book. I usually take an hour or two to meal prep every Sunday morning when Archer sleeps. I prepare lunch and my afternoon snack, and depending on what I think I want for breakfast that week, I'll prepare that, too.

Not only does this save me time after work every day, because all I have to do is take out the used food containers and pop in new ones, it also saves brain space. I don't have to think about what's for breakfast or lunch.

It also saves on food waste. As someone who lived off of $8 an hour in grad school while trying to make rent, food waste hurts my heart. I've made peace with having to waste food sometimes—I've had to in order to heal my last supper mentality and issues with food scarcity—but I still try to minimize it. If you just go into the grocery store and buy a bunch of food, not knowing how much you need or what you plan on doing with it, chances are a lot of it will spoil before you can eat it. Or you'll start eating things you don't want to just because you don't want them to spoil. When you do that, you won't feel satiated from your meals, which can set you up for overeating.

Another perk to meal prepping is that at least you can have nutrient-dense meals at the ready. I know that, no matter what, I have a yummy salad or power bowl ready to go for lunch in the fridge. If my colleagues randomly ask me to go to lunch instead, though, I don't feel obligated to eat what I packed simply because it was "the plan."

That hypothetical scenario, though, brings me to my next point: don't make meal prepping the reason you don't go out on a spontaneous lunch date with friends or colleagues. Meal prepping is done for convenience, not a rigid sense of control or fear. If you don't eat the lunch you prepped every once in a while, big deal. Maybe you can have it over the weekend or for dinner that night.

I distinctly remember one afternoon when my two colleagues wanted to go to McDonald's for lunch. I had just started working at my new district, so I wanted to make friends, but I had also packed a stuffed acorn squash for lunch. I was still a disordered eater, so I went to McDonald's ... but ate my acorn squash at the table. Looking back on it, I feel pretty embarrassed. They probably either thought I was really weird or just really rigid. I wish I had the flexibility then to just say to myself that it was okay to skip my planned meal and eat somewhere I typically wouldn't for the sake of bonding and camaraderie with my new colleagues. I'm sure I could've found something to satiate me; but you know what, I have to give that version of me compassion and grace and just be grateful for the fact that I'm not that person anymore. I'm proud of how far I've come since that day.

Transition Tip #8: Portion Out Your Food into Containers

I'm proud of you if your diet culture alarm just went off. It should've. Typically the words "portion" and "containers" are diet culture's way of restricting us and putting us in a box by thinking everyone should be eating the same amount or that one person should be eating the exact same amount every day.

Instead, become curious about how much, on average, it takes to keep you full and satiated. You know your body better than those who create the container programs and online calorie calculators. Offer yourself a serving of whatever you enjoy eating, and see how you feel. If you are full before you finish, you can stop. If you want more, there's no guilt or shame in that. Some days our bodies require more energy than others. It doesn't mean something is wrong or that you shouldn't be eating more. Listen to your body.

Portioning out into containers while meal prepping also ensures that you have equal portions for breakfast and lunch each day.

Transition Tip #9: If You Spend Most of Your Days Outside of the House, Pack a Lot of Snacks

I am the queen of snacks. I always have them on hand. People know they can ask me for food if they're hungry. Maybe that's the Italian mother in me. I know that if I go too long without eating, I will end up binge eating, because I'll be past the point of comfortable hunger and just want to shovel things in and around my mouth. I also know I will feel anxious, because I will feel the way I did when I was restricting. To combat those feelings, I always keep a variety of snacks in my purse. My go-tos are nonperishable protein sources like protein bars or turkey jerky. Sometimes I need them because my oil change is taking longer than expected; sometimes it's because what I packed for lunch wasn't enough, and I want to honor my hunger.

In addition to packing snacks in your purse, pack them in your lunch bag. I never know what type of afternoon snack I'll be craving when the "two o'clock slump" hits. Maybe it's yogurt and an apple with nut butter. Maybe it's a homemade nut butter bar with jelly. Maybe it's dates with a side of carrot sticks and ranch dressing. Maybe it's hard-boiled eggs with a protein bar. I'll pack several of these combinations and make a game-time decision when my tummy alerts me it's time to eat.

So far, we've discussed physical hunger and taste hunger, but this type of forethought honors another kind of hunger: practical hunger. Sometimes, because we're all so busy, we have instances where we have to go hours without eating, and in order to prevent a binge, we eat before this long stretch of time, even if we're not hungry. For example, sometimes I teach three hour-long classes in a row. I may not be hungry right before that first class, but I know that if I wait until after the last class, I will be light-headed, irritable, and not in tune with my bodily cues. This is acting in a practical way that honors your body and what you know of its needs.

Transition Tip #10: Regain Empowerment

As you'll hear a lot in this book, many of us became disordered eaters because we were looking for a sense of control. We feel out of control in our lives, so we try to take control of our food, our caloric intake, and our bodies.

While this type of control isn't very healthy for our mental well-being, we can exercise some empowerment over our food without feeling restricted. Here are a few hacks to take back some of that power without sacrificing your mental health.

First, you can cook more! Not only can cooking be a very relaxing hobby, but you're also learning something new. Challenging our minds and skill sets is never a waste of time or energy. When you cook at home, you have control over the ingredients. When we go out to restaurants, they tend to cook with a lot of salt, fat, and sugar. In fact, a recent study showed that people underestimate how much sodium is in restaurant food by 600%.[30] Not that ingredients like salt, fat, and sugar should be avoided or feared, but we can make meals that are just as delicious at home and decide for ourselves how much of these ingredients is enough to still make a delicious meal. Would I recommend skipping oil in making vegetables altogether because fat will make us fat? Absolutely not! Would I advise throwing a fistful of salt into them and drowning them in oil? Also, no.

That brings me to my second tip: Use an oil spray instead of a bottle of oil. Not only does this help you control the amount of oil you put on veggies or whatever you're cooking, it gives you more even distribution than if you just free-hand pour it over your food.

My last hack is putting sauces and dressings on the side. That way, you have power over how much you get on every bite. There's nothing worse than overestimating how much dressing you need on a salad, because by the time you get to the bottom, you have a soggy, overpowered mess. You also can't taste the fresh ingredients of the salad if

30. Alyssa J. Moran, Maricelle Ramirez, and Jason P. Block, "Consumer Underestimation of Sodium in Fast Food Restaurant Meals: Results from a Cross-Sectional Observational Study," *Appetite* 113 (June 2017): 155–61, https://doi.org/10.1016/j.appet.2017.02.028.

you're overpowering them with dressing. Keep in mind, though, this is not an exercise in how little sauce or dressing you can get away with using. You should be dipping or pouring as much as you want, but the point is you're "customizing" your eating experience to what feels and tastes good to you.

Transition Tip #11: Thicken and Protein-Boost Your Homemade Sauces

Again, we're not looking for hacks and swaps where the alternative tastes nothing like the original and leaves you feeling unsatisfied. Don't get me wrong, I love a good vegan macaroni and cheese sauce made with nutritional yeast, but I'm also not delusional enough to believe the vegan cheese sauce tastes like actual dairy cheese sauce.

As I said in a previous chapter, intuitive eaters aim to have authentic health and approach food through an abundance mindset. If you're looking to, for example, add more protein to your meals, find ways to do it that feel fun and satisfying, not daunting and obligatory.

One tried-and-true way that I add extra protein to my diet is by adding collagen powder. If I'm having a protein shake for breakfast, I'll put a scoop in. It provides me with nine extra grams of protein and a full amino acid profile. It also helps to thicken up my protein shakes. If I'm not having a shake for breakfast, I'll add it to my morning coffee because it's flavorless.

My second protein hack is uilitizing plain Greek yogurt. My favorite way to use it is by stirring it in adobo sauce, which is perfect for spicy, Mexican-inspired meals. Still, sometimes this hack doesn't cut it, so it's a game of trial and error. When I make black bean burgers, only good ol' fashioned mayo will do; when I tried the Greek yogurt sauce with the black bean burgers, I just felt like something was missing and found myself wanting mayo. We don't want those thoughts and feelings when we're eating intuitively! Not finding options that truly satisfy us only leaves us grazing foods, until we eventually find ourselves overindulging on what we originally wanted.

Another way to use plain Greek yogurt, as I said before, is in place of sour cream. As with the adobo sauce, this works best with hot and spicy meals that would normally include a dollop of sour cream on top, like chili.

My last thickening protein hack actually comes by way of my husband, Scott, when he was in charge of making vegan mac and cheese one night. Normally, I would thicken the sauce the traditional way: with flour. While eating that night, he asked me if I noticed anything different. I didn't; it was as delicious as any other night.

That's when he told me he thickened the sauce with unflavored pea protein powder. I was blown away. I would've never thought to do that! Ever since then, I've used pea protein to thicken sauces like curries, chilis, and chicken pot pies. Trial and error! Have fun with it!

Transition Tip #12: Stay Hydrated with a Stainless Steel Water Bottle

Diet culture tells you to drink a glass of water to fill you up so you eat less food and lose weight. Instead, drink a glass of water because hunger is often confused for thirst. Maybe you really are just thirsty; then again, maybe not. But treat it as an experiment. *Hmm, am I thirsty? Let's see ... nope, I still feel hungry. Okay, let's eat.* The same philosophy from the first strategy also applies here: You don't want your car to break down on the side of the road, and as you wait two hours for AAA to show up during a heat wave, you become dehydrated. Dry mouth and a thirst headache are just about as fun as a broken-down car.

I personally choose a stainless steel water bottle because plastics have been "linked with severe adverse health outcomes such as cancers, birth defects, impaired immunity, endocrine disruption, developmental and reproductive effects etc." [31] It's better to leave a stainless steel water bottle in a hot car than a plastic one. Plus, they're more environmentally friendly, economical, and durable. And let's face it, they're prettier; you can get them in all sorts of sizes and colors to fit your personality.

Transition Tip #13: Set It and Forget It with a Slow Cooker

By far, my favorite bridal shower gift was my Wi-Fi-enabled slow cooker. This was back when I was commuting an hour to and from my previous school district, and I knew that from the time I left to the time I got home, I would be out of the house for eleven hours. Even though you can't really overdo a meal in the slow cooker, that's a lot of time, even if you set your device to "low." With the Wi-Fi-enabled slow cooker, I was able to change the settings from work.

Even if you have a traditional slow cooker, all you have to do is dump the ingredients in and turn the dial. Just a little planning and prepping can make it so you have delicious, nutrient-dense foods already made for the week. This self-care is just another way to send yourself the message that you and your body deserve to be taken care of, instead of just taking care of everyone else.

Transition Tip #14: Go to the Grocery Store with a Full List and a Full Belly

If you go to the store with your list as your mission, you're less likely to deviate from it; and while I'm also all for giving into cravings, I

---

31. Neeti Rustagi, S. K. Pradhan, and Ritesh Singh, "Public Health Impact of Plastics: An Overview," *Indian Journal of Occupational and Environmental Medicine* 15, no. 3 (2011): 100–103, https://doi.org/10.4103/0019-5278.93198.

have a lot more cravings when I go to the grocery store starving. It's the difference between getting five different pints of ice cream because my eyes are bigger than my stomach, instead of one pint of ice cream that I truly had my eye on.

It's really important that when you implement these strategies that you remember that intention is everything. These same tips and tricks can be used in disordered ways to further your dieting and weight loss efforts, but that's not why I shared them with you. They are ways to keep you feeling good in your body and exercise gentle nutrition, without restricting or sacrificing satiety, both of which will only lead to erode the trust we have with our bodies.

Transition Tip #15: If You're Cooking-Averse, Ditch the "Wellness Culture" Version of Cooking

Many people fall into the wellness culture fantasy: the one where they only buy fresh organic foods with clean ingredients and have hours to spare to expertly prepare beautiful, Instagram-worthy meals completely from scratch. Even their snacks are prepared in pretty mason jars on a huge, marble-topped kitchen island, surrounded by an enormous and gleaming-white kitchen.

Hard pass. Did I mention I have a full-time job, my side business, and my toddler yet? I don't have time for this. Not many of us do, and that's okay. I'm giving you permission, here in black and white, to utilize convenience foods. Almost all of the vegetables I eat are from frozen bags. I also use a lot of frozen fruit that I bought in bags from the freezer aisle. I love instant oatmeal, precut vegetables and fruits, frozen veggie burgers, frozen chicken tenders, and jarred marinara sauce, the last of which might get me in trouble with my Italian family, but I am who I am. That's not to say I can't make my Nana's marinara sauce, but it's just not realistic all the time.

Using convenience foods doesn't mean you're not nourishing your body or that you're not eating healthfully. It does not mean you're cheating somehow. Many of you want to do everything perfectly and by yourself to show your worthiness, but it's not necessary. Use convenience foods to free up more time for other things in your life that you enjoy. It's okay to cut corners and to maybe give B- work sometimes if it means the balance of your life is sustained and that your life is rich with many things in it.

Of course, convenience foods can vary in quality. See which ones feel good in your body and which don't. Remember that if you have two options, and they both will leave you feeling satisfied, it's okay to choose the one that is traditionally viewed as healthier. For example, I do try to be mindful of how much sodium is in some frozen foods, but I will never choose one over the other if the "healthier" option truly won't leave me feeling satisfied. Fortunately, there are many brands to choose from, so you can experiment and decide which brands leave you feeling nourished and satiated.

CHAPTER 7

Setting Boundaries with Yourself and Others

Isn't it interesting how we find it harder to set boundaries with the people we're closest with? The people that we love the most, trust the most, open up to the most—and we don't feel comfortable being honest with them about our needs during recovery. Perhaps you're afraid to lose that person or for them to perceive you differently. You fear somehow losing that person because you are speaking your truth.

One of the things to keep in mind here when setting boundaries is that anyone's issues with your needs in recovery or inability to provide you with support are a direct reflection of their own thoughts, not you as a person. For example, if someone makes a comment about your weight when they see you for a family gathering, it's coming from their own beliefs about weight, probably including fatphobia. Weight, on some level, must equal worth to them, and that's their problem, not yours. If they're commenting on the fact that you're actually eating a hamburger *with* a bun at the annual family cookout, that comment has everything to do with their own faulty diet culture beliefs and nothing to do with your worth or morality. All comments given to us are neutral; it's what we make them mean that causes us to feel fear and shame around food and our bodies.

This is, perhaps, one of the most vulnerable journeys you will go through in your life. You're openly admitting you have a mental health problem; it might even present itself like an addiction if you can't stop bingeing, body checking, or dieting. Addictions, disorders, and mental health—despite many initiatives to eradicate stigmas—still carry a lot of shame for many people.

Obviously, this shame is a primary reason I'm writing this book. There shouldn't *be* shame around mental illness because *no one* is perfect. I would wager that almost everyone has some form of mental illness; everyone has inner demons. If we were all a little more open about our struggles and journeys and willing to share our strategies for recovery with others, the world would be a more connected, en-lightened place.

Why Boundaries are Necessary for Recovery

It's a sad reality that most of the world has adopted the language of diet culture. Since recovery is as much about mindset as behavior, you need to closely monitor the narratives you allow yourself to express, hear, and internalize. If you can minimize diet culture's narratives and replace them with ones centered on body and weight neutrality, it will be much easier to achieve long-term recovery.

When you monitor the narratives you take in, you feel empow-ered. You feel a sense of power over the language you hear. Just as it's important to be mindful of what foods you ingest, it is also vital to be mindful of the *messages* you "ingest." The messages you hear most often are what you internalize, and therefore, believe. Maybe that's how you got to where you are today in the first place. Maybe you wouldn't be disordered with food if your mom wasn't constantly off to diet meetings, and dragging you with her, or only drinking weight loss shakes when you were young and impressionable. Maybe you wouldn't be disordered if you weren't an avid reader of magazines that splay headlines like "Lose 5 Pounds in 5 Days," "A Flat Belly in One Fast Move," or "Get Slim at Any Age." Maybe you wouldn't be disordered if you didn't have friends who were cutting out carbs, counting calories, and talking about how fat their thighs were when you all were in middle school.

It's all around you, your entire life; it's really no wonder you've taken on these ways of thinking or even believe them to be facts. But you can take the power back when you selectively decide what you are willing to hear.

Filtering others' narratives also allows you to naturally avoid triggers. A trigger is anything that causes a negative emotional reaction. Triggers can make you feel angry, sad, frustrated, hopeless, anxious, or otherwise unsafe. By keeping diet culture's lies at bay with boundaries, you can minimize your risk of being triggered and experiencing setbacks in recovery.

Without all this talk about diets, weight, and body parts, whatever will you talk about!? The good news is that the opportunities are actually endless. There are many in the intuitive eating space who believe diet culture was created by the patriarchy as a way to keep women distracted with trivial things like bodily aesthetics, so that men could continue ruling the world. And just to clarify, the word "patriarchy" isn't synonymous with "men"; I mean people who support a society that disproportionately *favors* men over women. Men are not the problem; a patriarchal society that doesn't appreciate and empower women is the problem. Based on how much brain space my disorder took up, it doesn't sound too far-fetched to me. If women are too busy worrying about their bodies and whether or not they're desirable, they don't have time to change the world or use their time and energy on things that matter; not to mention, your energy is severely depleted and you have brain fog when you're restricting.

And that is certainly not to say that men are not affected by eating disorders. In some ways, it's even more difficult for men who suffer, because it's more socially acceptable for women to have eating disorders. According to society, men are supposed to be mentally and physically strong; there is no room for weakness or emotion. Some men experience dysmorphia, since the ideal body type for a man is equally as unrealistic as for a woman. They are told they should have bulging biceps and six-pack abs, and those things require a very specific and rigid eating regimen combined with hours upon hours at the gym. Attempting such strict protocols could put a man in the same binge-restrict cycle as a woman. When the "clean eating" becomes too much to bear, it can result in the same binge and the same residual shame that a woman would experience.

None of us, no matter how you identify, is exempt from the rules and expectations that society puts on us.

The People Who Need Boundaries

Again, the people around whom you may need to create the most boundaries are those closest to you. These people may feel comfortable enough, or perhaps even entitled, to have no filter in their conversations with you, and that includes any conversations they want to have about food and body. Typically, women in your family and your closest girlfriends will be the people you want to start creating boundaries with first. I find that family members typically will make comments that appear more critical in nature. It may be coming from a well-meaning place; maybe they are trying to point out perceived "flaws" so that you can "fix" them and reduce the risk of pain/rejection/shame later. Even though I usually say intention is everything, this criticism is damaging and triggering, regardless of intention.

With girlfriends, though, I find that diet culture messages infiltrate the conversation from a place of camaraderie and commiseration. If one girl talks about how fat her thighs are, one of two responses is expected. The first is, "No they're not fat. You're beautiful!" which is damaging because it suggests that being fat and being beautiful cannot exist on the same plane; the second is, "Oh my God, not as fat as mine!"

That's not to say well-meaning coworkers might not tell you how "great" you look if you've lost weight or talk about how they wish they could lose weight. Setting boundaries at work can be difficult in a different way, though, because we don't know those people as well. Setting boundaries can come across as rude or may make the commenter feel defensive. We have to eventually become okay with people not liking us or understanding our journey, but this can take some additional mindset work.

Even if what is said is well-meaning or meant to be taken as a compliment, we have to dive into why we are seeing those comments as such. When people would "compliment" me about how thin I looked, it only made me want to lose more weight. These people had no idea how disordered my behaviors around food were and that their well-meaning compliments only served to perpetuate my sickness. We never truly know what someone is going through, so when we criticize or compliment someone on their body, we can unintentionally praise or perpetuate unhealthy thoughts and behaviors.

If they're not commenting on *your* body and appearance, they might be commenting on their own. *They* need to lose weight, *they* have a big butt, or *they* need to go on a diet to lose the ten pounds they gained during the holidays. Those comments can trigger comparison culture: If they're so worried about the size and shape of their butts, should you be worried about the size and shape of your butt, too?

Aside from those around you, you need to filter the narratives of the voice *inside* of you, the food police. I already discussed in the introduction that the food police is the voice of diet culture that has found a home within your conscious, and even unconscious, thought. It's important to note, though, that this voice is separate from you; you are not your eating disorder voice or your food police. This realization makes it easier to separate and eradicate this voice.

How to Set Boundaries with the Food Police and Those around Us

There are some effective ways to set boundaries both within yourself and for those around you. There is room for experimentation here, too, as you know the people in your life best and what type of message to which they'll be most receptive. With that in mind, here are several tips you can mix and match. See what works for you!

Boundary Tip #1: Write Down What Your Triggers Are and What Type of Talk You're Not Willing to Tolerate

Triggers are different for everyone. When it comes to social media, different posts trigger different people. I'm not personally triggered by the "what I eat in a day" posts. I don't find myself comparing what I eat to what others eat and feeling guilty about my food choices. Before and after photos, though, can be triggering for me. Should I feel bad if my body looks more like their "before"? Should I strive to look like their "after"? Should I feel guilty if I don't want to make a transformation at all? Look through your social media and be cognizant of how you feel when you see certain posts. If you don't feel good about yourself when you see these posts, that's an indication that those posts are triggering for you. You can unfollow accounts that post that type of content.

For potentially triggering face-to-face conversation, prepare by writing down what kind of talk you will not tolerate. Insults should be the first on the list. No one should be insulting you, including you!

Moving away from the obvious, how do you feel about compliments regarding certain body parts? Your weight? How do you feel about conversations that include numbers? Is discussing weights, calories, or macros triggering? What about diet conversations? When someone talks about cutting carbs, does it make you feel that you should, too? If they talk about how they shouldn't have eaten a slice of pizza, does it make you feel like you don't want pizza? These are indications of conversations you want to no longer be a part of, particularly if you are in recovery. Even the compliments: if you are seemingly okay with those, it might be worth challenging why they mean so much to you, as this can indicate some mindset work that needs to be done around self-worth and fatphobia.

Writing different topics and scenarios down is helpful in terms of being clear and concrete with the boundaries you want to eventually establish. Now that you know *what* boundaries you want to establish, let's talk about *how*.

Boundary Tip #2: If the Discussion Is Happening as Part of a Larger Gathering, It's Totally Acceptable to Just Walk Away

If you're at a party, no one is going to be the wiser if you walk away to "use the bathroom" or "grab a drink." This strategy is for those who know they need to filter the narratives around them but aren't necessarily ready for actual confrontations. Quietly excusing yourself is absolutely acceptable. If you're at a dinner table and the people to your left start talking about diet-related things, physically turn your body to the right and see what those people are talking about.

Boundary Tip #3: Don't Get Combative or Defensive

Sometimes, especially if someone is being critical, you want to come back with fighting words. *What does THAT mean? Why would you say that?* But we don't want to be defensive because that puts people's guards up, and then no one is really hearing what anyone is saying. It shuts down meaningful, productive conversation instead of facilitating it. Part of the reason you may get defensive is because, deep down, you still believe diet culture's lies, too; and in that case, it's not exactly fair to go into attack mode. They, like you, are a casualty of diet culture's messages, and the fact you still believe diet culture's messages, too, is not their problem—it's yours.

Boundary Tip #4: Write Down Your Responses Ahead of Time and Be as Honest as You Comfortably Can

You already know the people in your life and the typical diet culture narratives to which they subscribe. You already know your friend Karen has issues with her weight, and Stephanie is always trying the new fad diet, and Rachel has her own disordered eating habits she doesn't even know about but always obsessively counts her macros. Write down what you think future disordered conversations with them will be like based on your past conversations. What will they say and what will you say back? Again, writing things down helps us get clear on what we want and don't want in the narratives we speak and hear. You can feel more confident in your responses if you craft them ahead of time, and you won't stumble over your words in the moment. You want to say what you need to say with strength and conviction.

It's also worth mentioning that maybe you're not comfortable discussing your personal issues with someone in the workplace. Depending on who you're talking to, you might want to explain why you don't like diet talk. Still, it's amazing how many women have opened up to me about their body image and food struggles after *I* asked for boundaries around diet and body talk. It's remarkable how many of us share the same struggles but don't feel comfortable or confident enough to talk about them. If you are willing to discuss it, though, it might open the door for others to feel they can do the same.

Boundary Tip #5: You Don't Have to Be So Serious. Try Being Funny!

Although dismantling diet culture is serious work, you don't always have to be so serious about it! You can say something with a pun intended or keep it lighthearted with a bit of a laugh in your voice. This helps disarm the person to whom you're speaking, and they will likely be more receptive to what you're saying if they feel assured that your response isn't an attack. Here are a few examples:

UNWELCOME COMMENT: "You're going to eat all that?"
RESPONSE: "Yup, can't topple the patriarchy on an empty stomach!"

****

UNWELCOME COMMENT: "Have you lost weight?"
RESPONSE: "Yup, the weight of other people's opinions on my weight."

Anti-diet registered dietition and intuitive eating coach Jessi Jean has a really great "Love Your Body" podcast episode with a few more similar responses that are truly hilarious, yet effective.

Boundary Tip #6: Redirect the Conversation

This tip is really important to avoid potentially awkward exchanges. After you respond to their comment, quickly follow up by asking them about something non-diet related. Not only does that indicate that you're not up for discussing that topic anymore, but it redirects the conversation. It indicates that you still enjoy talking with them, but not about dieting.

Boundary Tip #7: Find Other Places of Support

It's very common for people to feel that their friends and family don't really "get it." Most people are unhappy with their bodies, strive to lose weight, and have unhealthy relationships with food. I certainly found that in my recovery, and even as a Certified Intuitive Eating Counselor, I don't think many people I have personal relationships with really understand what I do. If this is you, it may be beneficial to curate a support system online. Find people in the body neutral and intuitive eating spaces that align with the values you soon hope to embody effortlessly. Many out there are very willing to talk about their own experiences, listen to your struggles, and help support you.

Boundary Tip #8: Prepare to Let Go of Some Relationships

This can be a tough pill to swallow, especially if you're talking about family members or close friends. You may fear you are being "over-sensitive," that you should just be able to let things go, that it's not that big of a deal; but it is. Your mental health and happiness are *huge* deals, and you have every right to safeguard them, while asking others who supposedly care about you to do the same. They might not understand your journey, your requests, or how they themselves are wrapped up in diet culture, but they should still be willing to respect your requests.

If they can't do that for you, they're not meant to be in your lives in the first place. If talking about diet and weight is that important to them, perhaps they need to read this book, too. If they claim talking about these things is in the name of your health, you can kindly tell them that you're more concerned about your mental health than your physical health in this season of your life. If they can't honor that, then again, you have to question whether they truly care about your needs. That's not to say these people cannot come back into your life after you've healed, they've healed, or both, but people are meant to come in and out of your life. With food freedom comes a different phase of your life, and therefore different people who need to be, or not be, in it.

A final note on these strategies: Don't expect to do them once or twice and have them magically start working. According to more recent research, neural pathways (i.e., the way your brain thinks, your narratives, and your beliefs) take approximately four months to rewire, and that means constant practice and determination to change for the better. [32] This is why I say that you have to recommit to your "why" every day and set a concrete intention: you were slowly and methodically trained to think the way diet culture wanted you to, and now you need to give yourself the grace and self-compassion to slowly and methodically work your way out of it.

---

32. Tara Swart, Kitty Chisholm, and Paul Brown, *Neuroscience for Leadership: Harnessing the Brain Gain Advantage* (New York: Palgrave Macmillan, 2015).

PART 2

Reclaiming, or Newly Discovering, a Love for Fitness

CHAPTER 8

The Dangers of the "Perfect Body"

The second part of this book, in some ways, will sound like an echo of the first, and that's with good reason. The issues that plague you around food are echoed by the issues that plague you around fitness. You feel there is a prescriptive way to exercise, the way you feel there's a prescriptive way to eat. There is shame around doing it wrong and not having the correct physique as a result of doing it wrong. There are similarly deeper reasons for wanting to do it right to the point of obsession.

I also sound like a broken record to intentionally begin the process of rewiring your brain; you're welcome.

I'll start with one of my favorite mantras, which you've undoubtedly already picked up from the first part of this book: Intention is everything. Everything. You can have two people with the same behaviors, and their intentions can be totally different; and that is the difference between disordered and not disordered behavior. One woman can work out because she genuinely enjoys the challenge and strength gain; another can work out with the same weights, movement, frequency, and intensity, but do it because she hates her body and wants to punish herself for the food she eats and binges she experiences.

It's very important to be honest about who you are. You can tell anyone what your intentions are and make it seem as if you are not experiencing disordered behaviors, but only you know your truth. Only you know whether you need this book and other resources to help you heal your relationship with your body.

There is no perfect body. Think about it. Even if you look at a line of supermodels, they still all have different bodies. The shape and definition of their abdominals are different. Some have longer torsos and larger breasts while others have longer legs and bigger butts and even differently-shaped belly buttons. Even among the "conventionally perfect," there are variations in anatomy; and that's because our genetics vary! Two women could eat exactly the same, be the same height, complete the same exercise program, and still have different results. In fact, fifty percent of the response to cardio exercise is the result of genetic differences, according to a 2019 study. [33]

But, you may say, the common denominator with these women is that they're all thin, that you would settle to look like any of them. Yes, but the point I'm trying to make is that even among those who are said to have perfect bodies, those bodies differ, so which is the true perfection?

There's also a whole lot of photo and video manipulation happening not only with mainstream advertising, but also with social media photos, and even though you objectively know that, you still find yourself comparing your bodies to these photos or wanting to look like those people. We can't seem to disassociate what we see from what the truth really is. Most people on Instagram don't really look as polished as they appear. Many of them have taken literally hundreds

33. Robert Ross, Bret H. Goodpaster, Lauren G. Koch, Mark A. Sarzynski, Wendy M. Kohrt, Neil M. Johannsen, James S. Skinner, et al., "Precision Exercise Medicine: Understanding Exercise Response Variability," *British Journal of Sports Medicine* 53, no. 18 (March 2019): 1141–53, http://dx.doi.org/10.1136/bjsports-2018-100328.

of pictures of themselves to get just the right one. They're using additional lights. They're posing in specific ways. They have bronzer and highlighter on. They're using Instagram filters and Photoshop before posting. There's so much time and energy that goes into these photos, and the rest of us just expect to naturally and effortlessly look like them. It's impossible, even for them. Our standard is so high that it is actually not achievable by anyone! Our brains have a really hard time processing that, though. "Brain images are believed to have a particularly persuasive influence on the public perception," according to a 2008 study in *Cognition*. [34] In other words, our brains can't help but register what we see as truth.

I don't know if you're like me, but my response to that last paragraph would be: Well, when I go to the beach, I see a few ladies with rockin' bods, and last time I checked, you can't Photoshop my actual eyes.

Yes, that's true; but perhaps they just have conventionally accepted genetics. Some people do. Or, as is the more likely case, they are subscribing to diet culture. You don't know what really goes on in people's lives. What you see as the picture of "perfect health" might be anything but. You've been conditioned to think that health equals thinness; even many physicians believe that. But more and more research indicates that this is simply not the case. There may be a correlation, but that doesn't mean there's a causation between weight and health issues.

Moreover, let's revisit where this idea of perfection comes from. What's perfect for one person isn't perfect for another, so whose version of perfect are you even chasing? Is it yours? Society's? Your mom's? Your partner's?

---

34. David P. McCabe and Alan D. Castel, "Seeing Is Believing: The Effect of Brain Images on Judgments of Scientific Reasoning," *Cognition* 107, no. 1 (April 2008): 343–52, https://doi.org/10.1016/j.cognition.2007.07.017.

Many women I speak with worry that they won't find a partner at the size they're at, that no one will find them beautiful or sexy. The same goes for men. Speaking in heteronormative terms strictly for example, many men feel that women want a partner who is more muscular and stronger than them, a fit and glistening Adonis who can pick them up and whisk them away. Again, these are fantasies and ideas sold to us by the media. They only see thin, fit people with thin, fit people. Conventionally beautiful with conventionally beautiful. Not everyone wants that; it just happens to be what commonly sells whatever product is being advertised. I know plenty of people who prefer larger partners. One of my favorite recent studies confirmed this idea; a 2020 study with 150 participants showed that "women overestimated the thinness that men prefer in a partner and men overestimated the heaviness and muscularity that women prefer in a partner." [35] Plus, if you're worried that someone is going to judge your value as a person solely based on your looks, is that person even worthy of your love? Why would you want to be with someone who only values looks? Reversing that logic, is that the only thing you value in a partner? I would hope not. The values we want in a partner are the values we should be honing and appreciating in ourselves: loyalty, humor, affection, selflessness, intelligence, or whatever other traits you value.

Another thing to consider: Do you really want to be a size you're not meant to be, for your entire life, just for someone else's validation? That's like … holding in your farts forever because you don't want your partner to hear them. I'm sorry, but eventually they will hear them; they will smell them. And that's okay. That's human. Embrace your humanity. You're not a perfect cyborg. You are a wonderfully flawed, relatable human being.

---

35. Xue Lei and David Perrett, "Misperceptions of Opposite-Sex Preferences for Thinness and Muscularity," *British Journal of Psychology* 112, no. 1 (May 2020): 247–64, https://doi.org/10.1111/bjop.12451.

One last question to consider when it comes to trying to achieve that "perfect" body: What happens when you actually achieve it? Will you be more loved? Will you be happier? And if you think you will be happier, why is your happiness contingent on your outward appearance? Even without knowing you personally, I can almost guarantee that, even if you did reach bodily perfection, you wouldn't be happy. You'd want more somehow. Or you'd have taken such drastic measures to get where you are that you'd have crippling anxiety and pressure to maintain it. It's not all it's cracked up to be. Ask anyone who used to bodybuild. Follow Felicia Romero on Instagram or listen to her podcast. Read Madelyn Moon's book, *Confessions of a Fitness Model*. These people we look up to in terms of physique are miserable most of the time. Think about all the Hollywood stars who amass beauty, fame and fortune—and then take their own lives. Even if you have everything you think you want, those things will not bring you happiness. Happiness has to already exist inside you, and only you and your thoughts can cultivate it.

The Price of the Perfect Body

When I was at my lowest weight, I was my most unhappy. You would think I would be thrilled since that was my goal, however disordered, but I wasn't. I was constantly worried about the next day and whether I would gain back any of the weight. I was constantly thinking about food, cognitively impaired by the brain fog, weak from the lack of nourishment, and at the same time, I just wanted to be one of those girls who could go to dinner with her girlfriends, order what she wanted, and not think about the calories.

So can you achieve your version of the perfect body? You can. You totally can. But chances are, it will cost you big time. I can almost guarantee that the cost is more than you want to pay, whether you realize it now or not. I've discussed mental exhaustion already in terms of my own experience. When you're not giving your body enough sustenance, your brain can't function; neither can the rest of your organs, for that matter. It's the same if you let your car run on gas fumes. It's not going to run properly, and eventually, it will stop.

You end up hating your body more, not less, because you begin to resent the fact you have to work so hard to make it fit the mold you've created in your mind. You begin to resent your body for not bending to your, or diet culture's, will as easily as you hoped it would. Yes, weight can be manipulated, but weight is really just another part of your genetic blueprint. Going outside your genetically-determined weight set range is like trying to change your eye color or height. You begin to hate your body because you become fixated on what's wrong with it and the things you want to change about it, instead of focusing on the things you love about it and what it does for you. Putting a different lens on it, it's actually ableist to be so fixated on a few pounds. Are you able to use your limbs, walk, and move without extreme pain? If the answer is yes, then you are more blessed than many others.

For those who have been categorized as obese or morbidly obese and told to lose weight, you might not be at your natural weight set range because you have an unhealthy relationship around food. Intuitive eating is not a weight loss tool, but it could cause you to lose weight if your unhealthy relationship with food has been causing you to binge or overeat as an emotional coping. Will you still be in a larger body? Maybe. Will it be to the point where you have trouble performing everyday tasks? Probably not. Will you have a flat stomach? Who knows? The point isn't the weight. The point is the relationship with food. Heal that, and chances are, you'll go back to your natural weight set point and alleviate whatever weight-related ailments you've been experiencing. If it doesn't fix your ailments, I would implore you to see a physician who supports Health at Every Size in order to get to the root of your health issues. Many intuitive eating coaches notice that when clients in larger bodies approach nutrition and fitness from a place of self-respect, they incorporate more nutrient-dense foods and more consistently move their bodies and *that* creates less mobility issues than the weight loss itself.

Many believe, though, that intuitive eating *can* be a weight loss tool because losing weight means being healthier, and that is simply a fallacy. Weight is only one small part of what makes up your overall health. Other things to consider are your overall nutrition choices, which don't directly correlate with your weight, your frequency of movement, your stress levels, your sleep quality, whether you smoke or do drugs, whether you have a support system, whether you feel you have meaning and purpose, your education level, your environment's pollution levels, your geographic location, your race and ethnicity, your genetics, etc.

In fact, the obesity paradox is a scientific hypothesis that suggests being slightly overweight actually leads to increased longevity, compared to those who were categorized as normal weight, underweight, or obese. [36] There are several factors that may contribute to this correlation, including that overweight people tend to receive more medical care or because those extra pounds help to cushion bones and organs.

Speaking of health issues, being under your weight set range can also contribute to health issues, including fragile bones, fertility issues, hair loss, anemia, and a weakened immune system. Your goal might be weight-centric, but that doesn't mean other areas of bodily function won't be affected.

---

36. Katherine M. Flegal, Brian K. Kit, Heather Orpana, and Barry I. Graubard, "Association of All-Cause Mortality with Overweight and Obesity Using Standard Body Mass Index Categories: A Systematic Review and Meta-analysis," *JAMA* 309, no. 1 (January 2013): 71–82, https://doi.org/10.1001/jama.2012.113905.

You can form different types of eating disorders, as well; just because you have the symptoms of one doesn't mean you can't pick up others along the way. My five-year journey with disordered eating, as you read in my introduction, evolved from body dysmorphic disorder to orthorexia to binge eating disorder. They overlapped and fed into one another.

They also left me feeling very isolated. If my friends wanted to go out on a whim, I would get a lot of anxiety about going, or I would go and not eat or drink anything. If I didn't go, I would feel physically isolated. If I did go, but didn't partake in the libations, I felt socially and emotionally isolated. That's not to say that people who don't drink should feel isolated from their friends; my husband, Scott, has never drunk alcohol. But when you're not participating out of restriction and fear, you feel a disconnect from your friends who don't have these anxieties, hang-ups, and fears. You want to pack your own food to control when you can eat, what, and how much. You want to control where everyone goes to dinner so you can find something "acceptable." You don't want to share appetizers or dessert. You're not present in the conversations around you; you're thinking about the food you either had, "shouldn't have had," or wish you'd had.

Redefining the Perfect Body

If you're honest with yourself, you can admit that you've let society dictate what constitutes the perfect body. When you were born, you had no semblance of perfection, no body shame, no comparison culture to make you feel like you needed to change yourself. You had chubby legs and a round stomach. You ate when you were hungry and stopped when you were full. You didn't wish to look like another baby. That would be ridiculous. So where does this desire to be perfect and to be different come from? Society. The culture you live in. The messages you receive from others who have also been fed those messages.

Geography and time have shown us that what constitutes perfection has changed over the years. At the turn of the 20th century, it was the Gibson Girl with the hourglass figure. Just twenty years later, it was the Flapper, whose figure was as straight as an arrow. Even between these two versions of the "ideal body," you can see how futile the mission to have the perfect body really is. There's no way a woman can be the Gibson Girl *and* the Flapper unless she plans on manipulating her skeletal structure. You either have long legs and hips or you don't.

We need to, as a body positive community, come together and say "no" to the unrealistic standards thrust upon us. We can only look like us. Our genetics are our family lineage, our history. The women in my family gain weight in their midsections, and that's just the way we are. I'm going to own that and proudly say I am a woman of my family. It is what it is, and it makes me feel connected to my family. There are all different types of bodies, and *you* get to decide which ones you find beautiful. You shouldn't let other people's perceptions of beauty dictate yours.

Look at yourself in the mirror. Not at your body but into your eyes. Try to look at your soul. *That* is who you are. Not your body. You are your love and your memories. You are not stretch marks and cellulite, although those help tell the story of your soul's journey in your particular body. I have loose skin around my belly button from my pregnancy with my son. I have stretch marks on my inner and outer thighs from preteen growth spurts. I have scars on my right oblique from an adrenalectomy. So what? Those tell my story. They make my body a road map of my experiences, and no one else's body can tell those stories but mine.

Confidence in Any Body

I've seen some conventionally beautiful women up close. Flawless skin, big eyes and lips, full shiny hair, tiny waists. I've also felt the lack of self-assuredness radiate from some of them. Shoulders slightly hunched as if to protect themselves from the outside world. Quiet. Eyes evasive.

And then I've seen other women who look very different from what society would deem physically perfect but have all the confidence in the world. They exude this vibe, this exuberance, this vivaciousness that is so infectious that I would rather be them over the insecure "perfect" girl. She doesn't seem like she wants to have any fun, but the other girl certainly does. The other girl is down for a cocktail. She's down to go dancing. She's not worried about how others perceive her. She is confident in who she is.

Instead of thinking about what you look like, think about how you show up. Are you standing straight? Are you looking straight ahead and into people's eyes? Are you laughing freely and speaking easily, with conviction and levity? That's what is beautiful: confidence, assuredness, a zest for life. That is what attracts people, be it partners or friends. That requires inner work and cultivating a love and appreciation for yourself. It does not require a certain pants size or number on the scale.

CHAPTER 9

Creating Your Fitness Goals
as an Intuitive Mover

We all have goals, and if you're reading this book, chances are you have or had goals for your body and weight.

As someone who values fitness, I understand you still have goals for your physique. We don't need to completely disconnect from those goals when we adopt the principles of intuitive eating. We do, however, need to get more specific about what those goals are and why we want them. Many of us just want to "be thin" or "lose weight" because that's what our eyes have been conditioned to deem as attractive. Those aren't ideal goals for authentic health. Authentic health, as defined by the founders of intuitive eating, is where introspective awareness, or being in tune with how our bodies feel, meets clinical guidelines for health.

First, and most importantly, goals fueled by a desire to be thin or a certain goal weight are ultimately not serving you. You don't actually want to be thin or lose weight; well, you do, but the *reason* those are your goals are actually not about your weight or your body at all. They go back to SALV: the need for safety, acceptance, love, and validation.

Secondly, those goals only serve to perpetuate the social narrative that thin is preferred, ideal, or superior. This narrative goes way past harming just you; it harms all those in larger bodies because they continually live in a world that caters to those in smaller bodies. As long as the thin ideal is alive and thriving, so is weight stigma and fatphobia for those who are not thin.

But Alana, what if I have an illness or my doctor says I need to lose weight in order to keep this condition under control? I'd say, most importantly, make sure you have a doctor who doesn't automatically suggest weight loss for your physical conditions. Causation and correlation are not the same thing. Let's say two people die on the same day, and they both ate bagels with cream cheese that morning for breakfast. Does that suggest it was the bagel and cream cheese that led to their deaths? There's correlation there, yes, but certainly not causation.

There is also an increasing amount of data in the scientific community that points to what's called the obesity paradox; we've been told for decades that fat is unhealthy, but increasing evidence points to the exact opposite. "Being overweight is now believed to help *protect* patients with an increasingly long list of medical problems, including pneumonia, burns, stroke, cancer, hypertension, and heart disease." [37]

Moreover, those goals of being "fit" and "thin" are too vague. What do they even mean to you? How would you even know when you've definitively achieved them? Vague goals are dangerous because there's no end to them, especially when your goal doesn't directly relate to your core need. My goal was to be as skinny as possible.

37. Harriet Brown, "The Obesity Paradox: Scientists Now Think That Being Overweight Can Protect Your Health," *Quartz*, November 17, 2015, http://qz.com/550527/ obesity-paradox-scientists-now-think-that-being-overweight-is-sometimes-good-for-your-health/.

Logically, I knew there'd come a time when, if I continued to pursue this goal, my organs would shut down and my parents would force me into in-patient treatment. But since I wasn't there yet, the goal still seemed viable. Once I reached a new low weight, though, I would push for even lower. When would it be enough?

Part of the problem here is actually goal setting itself. An 2016 article in *Forbes* reported, "Anchoring on a future goal triggers reward centers in the brain, inducing a cognitively soothing effect. That feeling of accomplishment becomes part of your day-to-day identity. You readily adjust to this new state of being so much so that actually attaining a goal turns out to be less satisfying than expected." So my goal weights would never be enough because I would need to keep getting skinnier and skinnier to feel the next "hit" of validation dopamine.

With vague goals, you don't get to enjoy the spoils of victory because you don't even know where you are headed in the first place. When you meet a goal in life, one that's worthwhile and made with positive intention, you find a deeper respect for yourself. You tap into a place of self-love because you set out to achieve something, and you accomplished it. You gain confidence, something that's vital in a food freedom journey. You want to set more goals, achieve more things for your one-and-only-life, and the cycle of positivity perpetuates. It's what finally breaks you from the negative cycle of shame and frustration that you've likely been experiencing.

As the Old Saying Goes: It's About the Journey, Not the Destination

Although achieving a goal is satisfying, it's not the most important part of a journey. There's always another goal, another mountain to climb. If we're done improving or striving, we might as well be dead. The achievement of the goal itself isn't the point because it's never the end. What matters most is who we are and who we become as we set and strive to achieve those goals. Are we making goals from a place of self-love and/or love for others? Are we punishing ourselves along the way if we don't consistently make progress toward those goals? Are we sacrificing other important things along the way in order to achieve these goals, like time and memories with friends and family?

When I was sick, I never wanted to go out to eat with friends two nights in a row. Never mind how lovely it was to have enough friends who wanted to spend time with me; I was afraid of too many cheat meals. What would that do to my progress toward being as thin as possible? I was denying myself nights of memories with my friends, all for numbers on a digital scale that don't even reflect actual health or happiness.

You might not even know what a more positive goal sounds like if you're a chronic dieter. I can't tell you what your fitness goals should be, but whatever they are, create them from a place of compassion and acceptance for your body; it doesn't have to be love, just as long as it's not hate or disrespect. As someone who is an ED-recovered intuitive eater, my goals are to feel strong in my body, to have great energy, to keep up with my son Archer, to balance my life in a way where fitness is only one passion and one part of my life, and to consistently appreciate it for what it can do instead of what it looks like. Although I would say most goals should *not* be related to aesthetics, this chapter *is* about setting fitness goals, some of which will perhaps be aesthetically related. If you know you shouldn't set a vague goal, but your goal is to have a six-pack because that's what society deems attractive and your means to get it are disordered, that's still not a positive goal to have. Not only should the goal itself be free from disorder, but the *means to get there* must also not be disordered.

Four Steps to Becoming a Better Goal Setter

Now that you understand why vague and disordered goals don't serve you, here are four steps to creating better goals that will more positively serve you.

Becoming a Better Goal Setter Step #1: Break That Big Goal into Smaller Goals

Let's say your goal is to run a marathon, which is over 26 miles. If you're not already "a runner," you have a long way to go. That's not to say you can't do it, but trying to tackle a goal that large can be discouraging. It can also lead to injury if you're not training properly.

Instead of thinking about running a marathon, think about running one mile. Check that goal off your list. Then two miles. You get the idea. Not only will this be a steady, safe progression toward your ultimate goal, but you'll achieve little goals, too, that boost your confidence along the way.

Maybe your fitness goal isn't a marathon. It's certainly not mine. I only run when I'm being chased. Maybe it's to hike a trail so you can take in that beautiful view. Maybe it's to get through a whole game of soccer with your kids. Maybe it's to take that ballroom dance class you always wanted to try, or be more confident in the spin class you've already been taking. A fitness goal doesn't have to be about body weight, aesthetics, or inches; it can be about strength, flexibility, endurance, mobility, and just performing daily tasks more easily. But those can be vague and large, if you don't get specific and break them up.

Becoming a Better Goal Setter Step #2:
Create SMART Goals

I do these with my high school students from time to time; goal setting for students can be crucial in terms of having them self-assess their strengths and weaknesses. A study by Gail Matthews, a psychologist from the Dominican University of California, showed that people who wrote down their goals were twenty percent more likely to achieve them than those who did not. [38]

You might have heard about SMART goals in grade school, too, but for those who haven't, here's a quick rundown. SMART is an acronym that stands for Specific, Measurable, Achievable, Relevant, and Timely. I've heard other variations of this acronym, but this is the version I've always used. We've already discussed specific goals versus vague goals, so we can skip right over "S" (for specific) and move onto "M." The ideal goal is measurable, meaning you can know, definitively, whether you've achieved it. Whether you're thin isn't really measurable, because that's subjective. We have to be careful with "measurable" goals when it comes to fitness and body because number-dependent goals can easily become disordered. I would say the "sweet spot" for measurable fitness goals are ones that have nothing to do with body measurements but are still measurable in a meaningful way. Maybe it's to not weigh yourself for *one* week. Maybe it's to increase the weight you use for bicep curls by *five* pounds.

"A" stands for achievable. You want to be realistic in terms of your fitness goals. Benching 300 pounds isn't very achievable for me. I wouldn't say it's impossible, but it's unlikely unless I have a true dedication to this goal. A more achievable weight training goal for me

---

38. Gail Matthews, "The Impact of Commitment, Accountability, and Written Goals on Goal Achievement," Dominican University Psychology Faculty Presentation, 2007, https://scholar.dominican.edu/psychology-faculty-conference-presentations/3/.

would be, within a three-week program, increasing my weights from twenty pounds to twenty-five pounds while squatting for one minute. The reason we want to pick achievable goals is so that we actually achieve them without disordered habits and feel a sense of accomplishment and gratitude for ourselves and our bodies once we reach them. This is similar to what educators refer to as the "zone of proximal development": the space between what the student can do on their own and what a student can do with assistance. You want to choose a goal that's right at the edge of what you think you are currently capable of so that you have to reach a little for it.

"R" is relevant. Are these goals relevant to your life? I find a lot of goals, like getting a six-pack, are formed through comparison to fitness professionals and social media influencers. One thought that has kept me firmly in recovery is, "I'm a high school English teacher." That's not to demean my job, because trust me, it's one of the hardest out there. Shout out to my fellow educators! It's only to say that it's not my full-time job to have the perfect body. No one is paying me six or seven figures to look a certain way, and that fact helps keep me grounded with my fitness goals. Do I want to improve my weight training? Yes, I love the challenge; but I'm also not going to spend six hours a day at the gym to achieve an aesthetic.

Finally, "T" stands for timely. Is this a goal that serves you in this season of your life? If you are recovering from chronic dieting that includes compulsive exercise, like exercise bulimia, maybe a fitness goal isn't the right thing for you right now. And that's okay. *Freedom with Food and Fitness*, and intuitive eating, is all about what's right for your mental health and your body, so don't feel discouraged if I'm talking about reclaiming a love of fitness and fitness goals and you're not there yet. You *will* be.

Timely may also mean putting a deadline on your goal, which helps you find the drive and determination to achieve that goal. I love fitness programs that have a definite beginning and end because I can create goals for myself within those weeks and see if I can achieve them by the end. They're never huge goals either, but I love setting and meeting those challenges. *Not* for the aesthetic of them, but for the achievement; although muscle gains and strength aren't terrible either.

Setting the goal, though, is only half the battle. Many of us can create strong and positive SMART goals, but we lack the consistency and follow through to see them to fruition. There are a variety of strategies that you can utilize to keep you on track.

Becoming a Better Goal Setter Step #3: Write Your Goal Down Where You Can See It Every Day

Write it in lipstick on your bathroom mirror, stick a Post-It on your refrigerator, create a graphic and make it your cell phone background. Recommit yourself to your goal every day when you wake up, and smile when you look at it—infuse it with the positivity it deserves because you've committed to doing something wonderful for yourself, out of love.

Becoming a Better Goal Setter Step #4: Get a Support System, Coach, or Accountability Partner

You *know* I'm forever here for you, and if you follow me on Instagram @FreedomwithFoodandFitness, then you already know you're part of my group. I answer every comment, every message. I'm a teacher through and through, and my life's mission is to help, coach, support, and teach others, whether they're ladies who want to finally achieve food freedom or students in my classroom.

It takes a village, though, and I'm not the only person who can support your journey. There are so many other fellow recovered women, dietitians, joyful movement coaches, and anti-diet advocates out there to inject your goals with empowering information and encouragement. Facebook also has great support pages and challenge groups. Get involved. Follow people of like mind. Comment on their posts and generate discussions that fill your soul and lift you up.

This type of support, especially if you're not getting any from the people in your life, is necessary. There are times on this journey to quitting diets that you will want to go back to dieting. You will get scared. The work will get hard and uncertain. You need someone with you, ideally a coach, who has expertise in the anti-diet space who can support and encourage you, while holding you accountable to food freedom.

Creating Fitness Goals

Now that you know how to set a proper goal, steps that you can use for any type of goal, what will your *fitness* goal be? Here are four tips to consider when choosing a goal specifically for fitness.

Setting a Fitness Goal Tip #1: Assessing Your Desired Workout's Intensity Level

There's a sweet spot between a program that's so easy that you're just going through the motions, and one that's so intense that you want to vomit halfway through each workout. At my current fitness level, I wouldn't do a prenatal workout, but I also know something like Shaun T's "Insanity" also isn't for me. That type of lightning fast, plyometric workout is too intense, and my body doesn't feel good or energized when I'm finished. My suggestion is try a few different kinds of exercise: swimming, running, yoga, cycling, etc, and see what feels best to you in terms of intensity. Or if you, say, really like yoga, take a few classes at different intensity levels to see what feels best.

Setting a Fitness Goal Tip #2: Assessing Your Current Level of Fitness

This goes hand-in-hand with the previous tip. If you're just starting out, don't try something too intense. Not only are you going to feel wiped, you also risk injury. If your body simply isn't ready for something in terms of strength, endurance, flexibility, or mobility, you set yourself up to fail that goal. You want to make sure that you're not, on some level, choosing things that are too intense as some sort of self-fulfilling prophecy either. You may choose a program that is too intense for you; and once you're unable to keep up with it, you may hear thoughts like, "I *knew* I couldn't do it. I'm worthless."

Setting a Fitness Goal Tip #3: Assessing Physical Limitations

Even though I'm in decent shape and exercise often, there are still certain moves I avoid, particularly certain exercises that require me to balance while kneeling on one knee. The women in my family have notoriously bad knees, and it's something of which I have to be mindful. If you've had injuries in the past, avoid programs that require you to work those parts of your body too often or too intensely.

Setting a Fitness Goal Tip #4: Setting a Realistic Time Commitment

Although you may be struggling with food and fitness, I have no doubt many of you are killing it out there. Whether you're a CEO or stay-at-home mom, our jobs are difficult, our hours are long, and we're being stretched in a million different directions. We don't have time to train like Olympic athletes, nor should we feel like we have to! With that being said, find a reasonable amount of time you can commit to fitness to reach your goals. I find that thirty to forty minutes of exercise, first thing in the morning, six days a week, before my husband and son wake up, works best for me. It's time I can consistently dedicate myself to my fitness, and when it comes to fitness goals, consistency is key.

Also be mindful to give yourself grace if you're at a season in your life where you can't commit as much time as me to working out. Even just fifteen minutes of exercise a day can lead to decreased risk of disease and increased risk of longevity, according to a 2016 study.[39] And isn't that the *most important* reason you should be exercising? Let's face it, we all don't have the same 24 hours in a day. Hollywood stars have nannies, personal trainers, and personal assistants while others juggle three jobs just to scrape by. The point is to find a consistent amount of time that works for your life and schedule.

Choosing fitness goals that make you happy takes honesty with yourself, a willingness to recommit to those goals every day, a dedication to checking in with yourself often to make sure they are still appropriate goals, and a whole lot of grace for yourself in your journey toward meeting those goals.

---

39. Jenna B. Gillen, Brian J. Martin, Martin J. MacInnis, Lauren E. Skelly, Mark A. Tarnopolsky, and Martin J. Gibala, "Twelve Weeks of Sprint Interval Training Improves Indices of Cardiometabolic Health Similar to Traditional Endurance Training Despite a Five-Fold Lower Exercise Volume and Time Commitment," *PLOS ONE* 11, no. 4 (April 2016): 1–14, https://doi.org/10.1371/journal.pone.0154075.

CHAPTER 10

Incorporating Movement ...
Gently and Easily

There are thousands of fitness programs out there, and they're solid starting points, but they might not be *exactly* what you need in terms of your fitness goals. They might not be challenging enough, or they might be too challenging; they might focus too much on cardio when you want to incorporate strength training, or vice versa; or they may be too long or short with regard to time. Again, gentle movement is finding a physical fitness routine that not only consistently fits into your busy schedule, but is also something you enjoy.

No matter how they may fall short of your specific goals and preferences, people tend to forget that they don't have to follow a program exactly as it's written in order for it to be fun and effective. That's really an idea fed to us by the diet industry, and many don't even realize it. You fall for the idea that you must follow an instructor who is telling you to do these exercises, this way, for this many reps, in this order, these days a week—or the program "won't work."

Gentle Movement Tip #1:
Know the Difference between Fitness and Movement

Movement can be exercise, but it doesn't have to be. Many times, in the intuitive eating space, we refer to "gentle movement" or "gentle fitness." This is the idea that we really just need to move our bodies in whatever way we enjoy in order to reap healthful benefits. Movement can be walking. It can be cleaning the house. It can be dancing around the kitchen while you cook. It can be bopping around with your toddler in the kiddie pool. Movement doesn't have to be "fitness," "exercise," or "working out" in the traditional sense. As long as your limbs are moving, regardless of intensity, you are doing something wonderful for your body.

I remember when I was in grad school, I would work out more the day after I binged, so typically on a Sunday, which was supposed to be my rest day. My most vivid memory of me needing to get in a workout after a night out was the day Hurricane Sandy hit New York. The night before, I had gone out with my girlfriends. We went to a carnival-themed bar and diligently sipped our way through the bar's signature five-gallon mixed drink (#teamwork); so suffice to say, my inhibitions around food were very much lowered. We ordered a bunch of appetizers to share: nachos, mozzarella sticks, avocado eggrolls, cocktail meatballs, all the typically off-limits stuff.

As I ate the food with my friends, the noise of their conversation and laughter seemed to mute itself around me. I wasn't contributing to the conversation with my friends. I wasn't laughing. I wasn't in the moment. It almost felt as if someone or something else took over my body, and I couldn't control how my hand kept going in for more and more food. I kept wanting to feel the sensation of food in my mouth and taste how delicious it was, because it was food I wasn't normally allowing myself. I didn't feel full because that's what happens when you drink; your brain stops receiving fullness signals from your body.

Finally, I snapped out of it and realized, with so much shame, that I had definitely eaten the most food out of everyone at the table. If, as a now intuitive eater, I ate more or less than a friend or my husband, I wouldn't feel shame over that, provided I was listening to my hunger, fullness, and satiety cues. But at the time, I knew I had binged because of my disordered relationship with food.

I honestly don't know whether I actually ate the most out of my friends that night or whether that was just something my eating disorder told me so that I could feel the shame it wanted me to. I also don't know if my friends had noticed that I was having a binge eating episode. Maybe I just felt it was as obvious to everyone else as it was to me. Regardless of what the reality of the situation was, I felt such deep shame for binge eating, for not having self-control or willpower, for not learning from the last time I binged, for not being present with my friends, for becoming a "food zombie."

The next day, I did a mental inventory of what I had eaten that night and tallied up how many calories I needed to work off; not only were these numbers probably inaccurate, given the intoxication, but I was also calculating them over and over, obsessively, for fear the numbers were wrong. Unfortunately for me, the college gym was closed because Hurricane Sandy was approaching. In fact, the wind had already picked up, and it had started to rain. I was so distraught by the fact I had overeaten and couldn't work out at the gym that I took a run outside … in the middle of a hurricane. That was one of the defining moments for me in realizing I had an actual problem. Going for a run in the middle of a hurricane isn't normal, as small twigs that had fallen off trees whipped around in the air and rain slapped me in the face.

Gentle Movement Tip #2: Incorporate Active Rest Days and/or Deload Weeks

A good litmus test for if you have a healthy fitness "why" is whether you're okay with this next strategy: incorporating rest days. Before I started my journey to recovery, I would work out every single day. I didn't feel that I could take a day off because that meant I would have to eat even less than the days when I did work out, because otherwise I'd gain weight. I didn't realize, at the time, that that idea was just a diet culture myth. I never gave my body a break, and as a result, I actually wasn't in great shape. My body was so weak from not being adequately nourished and not taking breaks from exercise that I really didn't have great endurance or strength. Disordered me would never be able to survive the type of exercise I can do today.

Now I make sure that I rest at least one day a week, sometimes two, depending on the intensity of the program. Typically on this day, I make sure I go on a walk with my son in his stroller and/or I spend a lot of time stretching every muscle I worked throughout the week. If I'm really sore, I'll make sure to use a foam roller on those areas. A foam roller is exactly what it sounds like: a cylindrical piece of foam that you roll over sore muscles to break up the facia, material that makes up your muscles, so they can heal quicker and stronger. If I'm feeling up to it, I will also do some light yoga.

Because I'm still incorporating movement into my rest days, they're referred to as "active rest days." I'm still moving my body, but I'm not challenging it in the way I typically do. The body needs rest from that type of intensity. When you work out with any sort of intensity, little tears form in your muscles. When the muscles repair themselves, they grow bigger and stronger, and that's how you see muscle gains. If you never let them go through a repair phase and you're constantly just tearing them, you're weakening the muscle, making the muscle susceptible to injury. Your bodies need self-care just as much as your mind does!

Similar to rest days and active rest days, deloading weeks are when you work out, but with much lighter weights and intensity. They give your body a chance to recover. Typically, these deloading weeks happen prior to starting a particularly intense regimen, so perhaps you don't need a deloading week if you're aiming for gentle movement, but it's an idea to consider!

Gentle Movement Tip #3: It's Not Just about Cardio

So many of my chronic dieters talk about this obsession with cardio because cardio is what will get you skinny. Yes, if you constantly do cardio, you'll burn a bunch of calories; but you won't be able to drag all your groceries into the house at once, that's for sure!

Do some form of strength training in order to build up your muscle mass. Muscle protects your bones as they weaken with age. It also helps you complete everyday activities. I have a toddler, and that little meatball is getting heavier each day. He also loves dancing with me, so I have to be able to hold him and bounce around for a few songs to satisfy him. I can't do that if I'm not strength training.

People usually think those are the two categories of exercise: cardio and strength training. Real athletes know there are two *other* key elements to true, long-term fitness: balance and endurance. You need core strength for almost everything you do in life, even getting out of bed in the morning. And I'm not just talking about your *rectus abdominus*, or your six-pack muscles. Your core includes your obliques (side muscles) and your back muscles, too. If you don't have good balance, you risk injury in everyday life. If you can deadlift 500 pounds, sure, I'm impressed, I guess, but if you can only do one rep, what good is that from a functional standpoint? Maybe you can run really fast for ten seconds, but can you sustain movement for thirty minutes without feeling like your heart is going to explode out of your chest?

Gentle Movement Tip #4: Alternate Muscle Groups to Give Them Time to Recoup

Alternate between cardio and strength training days. For example, on a Monday, I might do a cardio routine, then Tuesday will be an upper body day, Wednesday will be a lower body day, Thursday will be another cardio day, and so on. So not only am I alternating between cardio and strength training, I'm trying to make sure I don't strength train the same muscle groups two days in a row to give them time to heal.

Gentle Movement Tip #5: Don't Reinvent the Wheel

I don't want anyone sitting down with pen and paper to write their own workout regimens: exercises, reps, rounds, rest times, etc. I don't know about you, but I don't have the time, drive, or desire to do that. I'm not a fitness expert. I'm just someone who really enjoys working out and challenging myself, and I've been doing it long enough to pick up some basic, helpful knowledge along the way. I currently use at-home streaming services. I haven't stepped foot in a gym since March 2017, and I'm in the best mental and physical shape of my life. There are online programs for different ability levels, goals, and time commitments. Just choose one of those and tailor it to your needs. For example, for a long time, I hated any type of plyometric, or jumping, exercise, so while I was doing one specific program that included plyometric days, I would swap that workout for another one I enjoyed. There's no rule that says you can't do that. The fitness police won't come and take you away. Remember, the name of the game with fitness and intuitive eating is to do what you enjoy and forget the rest.

Gentle Movement Tip #6: Don't Listen to the Fitness Industry's Disordered Messages

If you're going to follow other people's workout programs, you're going to inevitably hear some messed up messages. Even businesses that offer varied, challenging, and well-structured fitness programs are, at the end of the day, still part of the diet and weight loss industry. They're going to promote diets and weight loss. We know better, though, right? So there are a variety of things you can do to filter that diet mentality from whatever workout program you're following. You can simply mute the TV and play your own music. You can print out and put body positive affirmations around your gym space while you work out; or my favorite strategy, which I do all the time because I'm sassy, is I talk back to them. If the instructor says, "Don't undo all the good you've done here in the kitchen," I tell them to shut up. Talk back to diet culture. Sass diet culture. Be empowered over diet culture while you get your sweat on, if that's what you enjoy! If that talk is still too triggering for you or you don't like the idea of even giving your money to diet culture aligned businesses, there are body inclusive options like Joyn, Big Fit Girl, and Yoga for Everyone.

Gentle Movement Tip #7: Don't Let Your Ego Get in the Way or Be Discouraged by Having to Modify

Honestly, I modify all the time, especially if I'm doing a really challenging program. I'm sorry, I can't do push-ups with a clap in between. I will break my face. I cannot do a whole minute of pull-ups. Some moves hurt my hips or my knees. I'm not going to injure myself or work until I feel I'm going to puke, pass out, and die. That's not fun. That's not healthy. It's okay to modify. It doesn't mean you're less than. Move your body because it benefits your overall health and it's fun. Once it's dangerous or a drag, it's not worth it because you're not chasing a body ideal anymore. You're not chasing a weight ideal anymore. You're not trying to be perfect anymore.

You also don't need to do whatever the modifier in the program is doing! Maybe that modification is too easy. Maybe it's still too hard. Remember, this is *your* journey, no one else's. There are a variety of ways to change the workout so it works for you: lose the weights and/or resistance bands, or replace the weights *with* resistance bands or vice versa. Lose the jumps in a movement and change them to pulses. Skip or step the move instead of jumping. Do fewer reps or do the movement more slowly. Or, as I did with my pregnancy, do a completely different move that works the same muscle group! When I was pregnant, I couldn't do any moves on my back or ones with twisting motions, so I had to get creative. Where there's a will, there's a way!

CHAPTER 11

Challenging Your Body in a Way
that Feels Good

Although you shouldn't abuse your body with fitness, if you have a positive fitness goal you want to achieve, you need to challenge yourself. There's nothing wrong with having fitness goals, nothing wrong with wanting to tone your muscles or get a bigger butt, as long as we're approaching that goal from a place of already embracing our bodies as they are. You're not dissatisfied with your butt as it is, but you're holding space for the goal of achieving a bigger one.

I accept, respect, and on most days, love my body. Of course, I have bad body image days, just like anyone else. I'm not impenetrable to the harmful and hurtful messages of diet culture, and sometimes I see these super fit and toned Instagram influencers and wish I could look like them, without an eating disorder; but on the whole, I look at my body, and I'm very grateful for the things it's been able to, and continues to, endure.

That also doesn't mean I don't have fitness and body goals. I can love the way my body looks right now but still work toward gaining muscle in my booty. Still work toward strengthening my core. Still work toward more definition in my arms.

But I'm not going to punish my body. It's simply a goal, kind of like I have a goal to revisit Napa Valley, better known as California wine country. It'll happen eventually, and I'll work toward saving up money to go when Archer is old enough to also enjoy it. It doesn't need to happen tomorrow, and I don't need to employ any drastic measures to make it happen, like taking out a loan to finance the trip. I feel the same way about my fitness goals. I have them, I work toward them, but there's no need to become obsessed and resort to drastic measures to get there. You will never hate yourself into loving your body.

If you feel you are in a place where you can approach fitness goals in this way, I can help you with specific strategies that will challenge your body and give you the results you want. These strategies can help cultivate body appreciation and trust. Although this book is broken up into two different sections, that's not to say that fitness and nutrition are not intrinsically related.

There are many that struggle with motivation to participate in movement consistently. Perhaps you're someone who has always had an all-or-nothing mentality; you're super intense at the gym for a few weeks, burn out, and then don't go back to movement for months. Maybe you have ADHD and find it difficult to stick to a routine. Those with ADHD often have trouble activating the use of executive functions in the prefrontal cortex of our brain; as a result, time management and motivation can be difficult. Maybe you're just discouraged by all the times you've failed to stick to a routine or to find movement you enjoy.

No matter the reason you've had difficulty with motivation, here are some tips for motivating yourself to stick to a consistent movement routine. First, physically block it out on your calendar. If it's on your to-do list, like anything else you need to get done, the chances of you getting it done are much greater. Put it on the calendar ahead of time, making a conscious commitment. Second, think about how your future self will benefit. Who do you want to be in the future? Do you want to be someone who is consistent with movement, who loves it, who experiments and explores with it, who uses it for authentic health and not unrealistic aesthetics? Then start thinking about becoming that future self. What would she plan to do? Would she follow through with her commitments to herself? You bet she would. The last tip is to throw out all the preconceived notions of what exercise is supposed to look like! It doesn't need to be an hour long; it's arbitrary wellness culture hoopla! We already established that only fifteen minutes a day, most days, is required for the majority of health and longevity benefits. Tell yourself you're going to do just fifteen minutes. Check in with yourself after those fifteen minutes. If you're not feeling it, you don't have to continue. If you are, you can go longer. Many times, getting the motivation to start is the hardest part. If you can promise yourself you can stop after fifteen minutes, the buy-in to begin seems like a lot less pressure. It also doesn't need to be intense! Simply gardening or walking is enough, as long as it's moving your body. Start small and start in a way that you can realistically and joyfully continue consistency.

Fitness can be considered a metaphor for life. You don't want to be obsessive or have a one-track mind about any one thing in your life. Do things that will benefit you not only in the short-term but also the long-term. Staying in shape and incorporating movement into your life promotes longevity, and what's more, longevity without pain. You can keep up with your kids and grandkids. You can participate in the physical activities that you enjoy: hiking, biking, walking, gardening, yoga, etc. It doesn't have to be deadlifting or something equally as intense. Seek to challenge yourself, not punish yourself. You only get one life, so strive to keep improving yourself, but from a place of respect for your precious life, not because you hate the person you are. Be consistent in working toward your goals, which is why I suggest finding a consistent amount of time you can dedicate to your fitness goals. When you really want something and commit to it as a goal, the only thing that will get you there is consistency. So let's talk about fitness challenges and consistency.

Fitness Challenge Strategy #1: Drop Sets

I love drop sets. They are a super effective and safe strategy for increasing weights. With drop sets, you complete half an exercise set with one amount of weight and the second half of the set with slightly lighter weight. This allows you to make a gradual increase in weights overall. If you're looking to increase your chest press weight from twenty pounds to twenty-five pounds, you can do drop sets for a few weeks where you do thirty seconds of chest presses with a heavier twenty-two pounds and then drop back down to the twenty pounds you're used to. Then, after a few weeks, you can start aiming for drop sets with twenty-five pounds (thirty seconds) that drop to twenty-two pounds (thirty seconds).

In the name of safety, I personally like to add an intermediate step. I will go from using twenty pounds for a full set one week, to a drop set of twenty-two and twenty the next week—but then I will take a few weeks to use *just* twenty-two-pound weights for the full set before I start doing drop sets of twenty-five and twenty-two. It gives me more time to get used to that intermediary twenty-two pounds before I make my way to twenty-five pounds. When you increase what you're lifting too much and too fast, your form suffers. Depending on the exercise, your back might start compensating for your fatigued muscles, your shoulders might start slumping forward, you might overextend your knee, or pinch a nerve in your shoulder. If you injure yourself, it'll take even longer to reach your goals because pulled muscles, at best, take several weeks to heal, provided you don't continue to injure them and need physical therapy or surgery.

Fitness Challenge Strategy #2: Track Your Weights

I work out with moderate intensity six days a week, around thirty to forty minutes a day. I do several different types of exercises when it comes to my weight training, and if I don't write down what I use from day to day and week to week, I won't remember. Did I use twenty or twenty-two pounds for my split squats last Tuesday? There's no way I'm going to remember that. I'm a full-time working mom.

I highly recommend tracking your weights when you are trying to make strength training progress; for those who are new to fitness, strength training is any exercise that includes weights or resistance of some sort (free weights/dumbbells, resistance bands, resistance loops, etc.). By tracking your weights, you can create goals, like SMART goals, for various exercises (squats, presses, etc.) over several weeks. Your goal doesn't even need to be super specific from workout to workout. A lot of times, my goal is to simply increase the weights I use for at least one exercise during the day's thirty minute routine. I don't need to increase my weights for every single exercise of my leg day. Maybe I just increase the sumo squats or just the calf raises.

It's unrealistic to increase every single time, too! And some days you're just not going to feel it. You're going to be more tired or have less energy, especially if you're menstruating. Don't feel like you're regressing, or the workout was a failure, or you're a failure. Give yourself grace, and don't forget, if you're increasing so much that you're risking injury or you're not having fun, you need to rethink your goals and your whys.

Between starting and finishing that last sentence, I actually ended up injuring one of my latissimus dorsi "lat" muscles, the large muscles in your back. I strained it by either picking up my son too quickly, lifting weights that were too heavy, or not using proper form for either. I won't be tracking my weights again until my muscle has healed, because right now, increasing my weights is the last thing I want to do. If anything, I'll be cutting what I typically use in half. I'll be icing my back and using physical therapy tape to support my back while it heals. I'm not upset at "the progress I'm not making" because the point isn't to look perfect; the point is to move my body and strengthen it as best as I can, but it's not the end of the world if I need to scale back for a few weeks.

If you're like me and not ready to increase weights for a while, ask yourself these questions to see if there are other ways to challenge yourself:

Can you do more sets?

Can you do more repetitions (reps)?

Can you increase your range of motion?

Can you put more power into the movement?

Can you put more speed into the movement?

Fitness Challenge Strategy #3: Get Comfortable Being Uncomfortable

Before I begin this one, especially in light of what I just said, there's a difference between being uncomfortable and being hurt or injured. If you feel like you're going to pull a muscle, fall, puke, or pass out, then slow down. There's no reason to push that hard. I don't care if you're training for a bodybuilding competition; although I sincerely hope you're not, because those can be just petri dishes of disorder.

That being said, there *is* a certain level of bodily discomfort if your goal is to challenge your body. Challenging yourself means doing something differently than you've done it before; this might mean faster, deeper, longer, or heavier. No matter the challenge, if it's something your body hasn't done before, you might feel a bit uncomfortable because it has to get used to this new intensity. Lean into it. Certain sensations of discomfort are normal, and you shouldn't be scared of them: muscles burning, heart rate increasing, breathing getting heavier, sweating. As long as you don't sincerely feel that you're going to do yourself harm, it's okay to feel a little uncomfortable. Know that it usually ends soon after the exercise.

This also goes for completely new forms of exercise that you're trying out. When I first tried yoga, even at the beginner level, I felt uncomfortable. The movements were different than I'd ever done before when I was a dancer. Just because I was uncomfortable at first, though, didn't deter me from continuing the practice and improving.

Fitness Challenge Strategy #4: Try a New Kind of Exercise

Challenging yourself doesn't necessarily mean taking the exercise you currently do and making it more intense. It can mean something completely different. As intuitive eaters who follow the ten principles, gentle movement includes finding movement you enjoy; that might require some experimentation.

I started incorporating yoga and Pilates into my fitness routine, which when I was disordered was 90% cardio. I started playing with volume training. I've tried ballet barre and mixed martial arts (MMA)-style workouts, too. Even try something you know you're not great at! I feel like I kind of suck at yoga, if we're being honest. I never feel relaxed when I do it because I'm always concentrating on not falling over. Maybe someone can give me lessons? I do like the challenge, though, and the breath work that goes along with it. I also like the stretching and lengthening aspect, so I stick with it.

Fitness Challenge Strategy #5: It's About the Little Things

There are so many small things you can do to challenge yourself more. Increasing mobility, balance, strength, and flexibility don't need to happen all at once. They happen through small increases over time, with consistency. It's holding a move for a few extra seconds in the form of what's called an isometric hold. Holding a move forces the muscles to work a little bit longer, under a little more tension. It's changing the "tempo" of the exercises and creating eccentric movement. An eccentric movement is when force is put on the muscle by moving slowly while the muscle is under tension. For example, you can do eccentric push-ups by quickly lowering your body to the ground and slowly pushing up using your chest and core muscles.

If you're someone who has healthy joints, you can add jumps to movements, especially lower body exercises (split squats, sumo squats, regular squats, lunge jumps, push-ups, etc.). Jumping or even a small hop increases your heart rate, as it turns the move into a plyometric movement that challenges your cardiovascular system and endurance.

If jumping isn't for you, try adding pulses to movements like shoulder presses or squats. Pulses challenge balance and muscles in a different way that's still time under tension. Resistance bands do the same! Add resistance bands to glute exercises. Create an element of balance by raising one leg in the air during bicep curls. That way, not only are you challenging your balance, you're also working on core stabilization, too. Simultaneously working multiple muscle groups is time efficient. Get in, get it done, and get on with your day!

CHAPTER 12

The Importance of Self-Care

There are so many metaphors I could use for convincing you that self-care is essential. You probably wear multiple hats—mother, father, partner, daughter, son, entrepreneur, employee, sister, brother—and are so busy cycling through these hats that you forget to wash the hair that's underneath. There, I created my own, kind of gross, metaphor just for you. It helps, though, to really bring home the point that self-care isn't selfish; it's necessary. Especially if you don't want to smell.

Some say that you have to "fill up your own cup" in order to nourish others. Others say, as they do on an airplane flight, "Put your oxygen mask on before your child's." What these all mean to say is that, despite your best efforts to do everything and be everything for others, if you don't take care of yourself, you can't effectively help others. You're only human. You're only one person.

What is Self-Care?

Self-care has become so trendy that the wellness industry has exploded to become a profiting machine. The image of self-care in the media is thin, happy women drinking $12 green smoothies with their yoga mats slung over their shoulders, while $150 lycra pants hug their taut bottoms. It's very focused on the *appearance* of the person practicing self-care and what they can buy with their money. That seems to send the implicit message that only those who are the "picture of health" deserve self-care because they've earned it through working and paying to look like that. Self-care in the media seems to also cater to the more socioeconomically advantaged. *Take these exercise classes, get this trendy massage or body wrap, drink these expensive detox drinks, and look cute in these over-priced sports bras.* Again, we have to be analytical enough to see through this facade. They are not selling health, wellness, or self-care; they're selling an ideal that they hope you buy into so they can take your money and profit off the fact you don't feel enough self-worth.

Real self-care, then, is anything that you do for yourself that is just for you. It's not to feel like you've checked another thing off your to-do list or another thing that will make you perfect or better in the eyes of others; it's something that feeds your soul, replenishes you, is fun, is relaxing, or is some combination of those things.

Five Kinds of Self-Care

Self-care is so personal in terms of what fills up someone's cup. I love to read. I always have. Some people are allergic to reading, and that's cool; even as an English teacher, I try not to take offense. Maybe they're into hiking, of which I've never been a huge fan.

Luckily, there are five different types of self-care. I suggest you find one kind of self-care that you enjoy in each category so that all the parts of you can be nurtured. Just as you don't want to focus on improving your body alone because it's only one, small part of who you are, you don't want to focus only on nurturing, healing, and repairing one part of your inner self either; self-care should be well-rounded. Keep in mind, too, that some of these can overlap and be placed in other categories. Hanging out with friends could be both social *and* emotional self-care. The particular category each activity falls into doesn't matter as much as finding activities that soothe your soul.

Physical self-care: For those who have fitness goals, this one is essential. If you come from a place of disorder, you may hate to take rest days because those are days you could be making gains or losing weight. I hear you. I've been there, too; again, though, if you don't allow time for rest and repair, you will do more harm than good in the long run. Ways to show yourself physical self-care can be an active rest day where you take a walk in nature, get a full eight hours of sleep, take a hot bubble bath, foam roll, lightly stretch, apply a clay face mask, book a massage or other spa treatment, or go dancing. There are dozens more, but those are just a few; and notice that I tried to incorporate some that come with a price tag and some that don't. Self-care isn't just for the financially advantaged.

Practical self-care: These are things that help organize or enrich your life from a pragmatic standpoint. As someone who is Type A, these activities calm down my brain rather than stimulate it. Maybe you want to create a budget. Take a professional development class, online or in person. There are plenty of free online courses you can take, some even from Ivy League schools. Maybe, instead, you'd rather grab a friend and take an in-person cooking class. If school isn't your thing but you're a fashionista, organize your closet. I'll admit I never got on the Marie Kondo train, but I do have a favorite closet organization hack: I make sure all my hangers are facing the same way, and I mark the date in my calendar. As I wear different outfits, I turn those hangers around. If, at the end of the year, there are outfits I didn't wear, I donate them to make room for outfits I'll actually wear. If you're like me and need to have everything written out or you'll forget about it, make a to-do list. Sit down and think about everything that needs to be done over the coming week. Put those things in order from most to least urgent and spread them out over the days of the coming week. That way, you know what needs to get done, that it's getting done in a timely manner, and you're not overwhelming yourself on any one day; that way, you can incorporate *other* kinds of self-care into those days, too!

Mental—emotional self-care: A brain that's always thinking is referred to as a monkey brain. Everyone's monkey brain sounds different, but chances are, if you're reading this book, your brain is on nonstop. Sometimes in order to reset it, you need to quiet it with mindless tasks. Maybe you're someone who likes to meditate. This can be with guided meditations, as there are a ton of free apps you can download to your smartphone, or just soothing music. There are also different meditation visualizations and techniques you can incorporate into your meditation practice. You can imagine inhaling your aura light and exhaling black smoke. You can do a body scan where you relax each part of your body, one by one, from head to toe. You can practice progressive muscle relaxation, where you clench each body part, one at a time from head to toe, and then release it, letting it relax. You can say "om" or repeat a mantra. Breath work also goes hand-in-hand with meditating, although you don't need to do it while meditating. You can do breath work any time of day when you need a reset or to be brought back into the present moment and activate your parasympathetic nervous system and calm the body down. Do this before you eat in order to aid in digestion. Studies show that experiencing stress and anxiety while eating can cause digestive and gut-related issues.[40]

---

40. Christine E. Cherpak, "Mindful Eating: A Review of How the Stress-Digestion-Mindfulness Triad May Modulate and Improve Gastrointestinal and Digestive Function," *Integrative Medicine* 18, no. 4 (August 2019): 48–53.

Journaling is another great way to get in touch with your emotions and mental state. Sometimes you don't actually know how you feel about something until you see it in writing, giving yourself a chance to dig deeper into your thoughts and connect one thought to the next. I see this book as one big journaling exercise for me. It's been very cathartic and reaffirming for me to work through some of my thought processes of recovery and to hear parts of my story again, to reflect on them for the first time since they happened, and see them through a retrospective lens.

If meditating, journaling, and breathwork feel too "woo-woo" for you, you can always use a hobby as social—emotional self-care. Read a book, do a puzzle, crochet. I would recommend doing something repetitive so that your brain can turn off. Heck, at that rate, watch something on Netflix! Find a guilty pleasure show to turn your brain off. I would totally consider that self-care.

Another form of mental—emotional self care is therapy. I know that, even by today's standards, there's a stigma around therapy. Only people who have deep-seated issues and are "crazy" go to therapy, right? Listen, Brene Brown—the queen of authenticity and vulnerability—has said she has a therapist. If she has a therapist, I think we should all have a therapist. If that's not an endorsement, I don't know what is. This is also a good time to remind you that, as much as I would like to think this book is helpful to someone going through recovery, this book is not a replacement for professional help. These were the strategies that helped me, and I'm giving you as much as I possibly can in the way of self-reflection, strategies, and advice, but there's simply nothing like having a licensed professional with whom to talk. With that being said, therapy can also be a form of social—emotional self-care. Talking to someone who is not only objective but also licensed to guide you through your mental health issues is paramount to recovery.

Social self-care: Social self-care is related to mental—emotional self-care. Social self-care is surrounding yourself with those who love you. Think brunch with friends, a date night with your partner, making time to regularly call or FaceTime your mom, cuddling with your favorite fur baby. Humans are social creatures by nature, and we seek a sense of belonging and communication. The former could very well be why you got stuck in the diet cycle in the first place; you want to feel like you belong, and you unfortunately live in a society where thinness provides that. The desire is evolutionary; when we were cave people hunting in packs, if we were ostracized from the pack, we would likely die of starvation or be eaten by a predator. Belonging was literally essential for survival. Obviously, things have changed since then, but the instinct to want to belong remains the same. Being around people who you know will provide that sense of love and belonging will help lessen that sense of needing to manufacture belonging through your body.

Being around people who align with the kind of person you want to be allows you to get out of your own head; of course, that time with people should be balanced out with introspective and rejuvenating time with just you. A large part of my recovery came when I moved in with my now husband, Scott. I wasn't living alone anymore, and I couldn't continue with the same disordered behaviors because I was ashamed of them. Having someone around almost as an unwitting accountability partner helped me get out of my own head and into the present moment with someone else.

Since basically everyone and their mom is steeped in diet culture these days, though, it's important to also note that while you want to surround yourself with people who love you, they may also be people who are toxic to your recovery. I have a few friends that are always actively trying to lose weight, striving to eat super clean, or speak ill of their own bodies. While I love these people to death and I know they would always support me, I know that spending time with them without first setting boundaries would be very triggering for me. If you need a refresher on setting boundaries, go back to Chapter 7.

Spiritual self-care: I'm not religious, but I would still consider myself spiritual. I think there's some kind of energy in the universe that guides certain things and people. Religion and spirituality can be very calming and healing. I love meditating. Others find yoga to be very relaxing. Walking in nature, even, can be a meditative experience. Perhaps you enjoy praying or just self-reflecting in a journal or sitting quietly in a dark room. Whatever it is, spiritual self-care brings you in touch with yourself and the energy of God or the universe. You can reflect, calm your mind, or allow space to be with your own thoughts.

How to Make Time for Self-Care

I know this is going to be the next question. Our schedules are always packed, and for many of us, if we're not being productive, then why are we living? As someone who has always struggled with making productivity and busyness a badge of honor, you can simply just capitalize on your Type-A organization skills and block the time out on your calendar. Share that event with your partner so they know it's nonnegotiable. You can even keep track of the time with the timer on your phone so you don't go over the time you've allotted yourself. When you're in that time, though, dedicate yourself to it fully. Don't be thinking about what needs to be done after or what else you can be doing with that time. Enjoy it unapologetically. Connecting with yourself in this way helps foster self-compassion and self-love. You are taking time to get reacquainted with you, checking in with yourself the way you would a friend or family member. The more we foster self-compassion and loving self-reflection, the more we will rely less on damaging and disordered behaviors or rely on our bodies for validation and self-worth.

Afterword

I've alluded to this a few times now, but physique and weight are not accurate indicators of health. We've talked about how inaccurate BMI is as an indicator of health. We've talked about the negligence of weight fluctuations. We've talked about the medical dangers of dietary restriction, overexercise, and falling outside your genetically-determined weight set range.

Your thoughts are not unequivocal truth. Just because you think something doesn't make it true. You have been conditioned to believe that thin equals happy, valuable, sexy, and safe. You are chasing this thin ideal because you've been told so many times that this is the truth and you've come to believe it. I can promise you though, weight loss is not going to get you a SALV(e); it's not going to get you safety, acceptance, love, and validation. The only thing that will get you those things is learning to accept who you are, learning to accept that society has created lies to increase its profit margins, and to accept that you were born having unconditional value, simply for being you. We live in a culture where we feel so compelled to improve all the time that we find it hard to believe that all of us, at birth, were born valuable and deserving of love. Everything else that we do is icing on the cake.

Even if we can say that eating more nutrient-dense foods will lead to longevity, we're talking only a few years; only in extreme cases would we really be talking decades. Eventually, all of us will die and go back to the earth. Yes, you can try to focus on the nutrient-dense foods you enjoy, but to force-feed yourself kale or restrict yourself to a 1,200-calorie diet meant for a toddler because you think it's going to buy you five more years of misery doesn't sound worth it to me. I'd rather fully enjoy a shorter life than torture myself with restriction and self-hate for a longer life.

I'd like to leave you with one last strategy, one that really helped put my issues with food, weight, and body into perspective; I call it "gravestone thinking," and it's based upon answering two questions.

"What Do You Want Written in Your Obituary?"

Do you want to be remembered for being loving, thoughtful, having a zest for life, being an adventurer, challenging and supporting others, loving with your whole heart, being present-minded, or being a good role model for those around you? Or do you want to be remembered as someone who fixated on her body and weight, who let the scale dictate her day, who never wanted to do anything that wasn't in her meal plan or conflicted with her workout schedule, who created an environment that made her children feel like they needed to achieve perfection, too?

"How Do You Want to Feel about Your Life on Your Deathbed?"

When you're lying in bed, hopefully at an old age, and taking your last breaths, what thoughts do you want to have about how you lived your life? Do you still want to be worrying about what you had for breakfast that morning? Do you want to feel like you wasted your life worrying about something that didn't even matter in the end? Or do you want to say, "Dang, I wish I could do that all over again because it was so much fun!"? A 2011 study revealed the biggest regrets of the dying. Inaction was one of them: Are you going to stay stuck in your dieting cycles because it's easier and less scary than the unknown of trusting and loving your body? Or are you going to take action? Other regrets were based on non-fixable situations. Your weight set range is written in your genetics and does not need to be fixed. So will you end your life realizing you were fighting a war against an opponent that didn't want to fight you in the first place? [41]

Your Life Is Yours, and You Only Have One

Ultimately, I can't tell you how to recover or whether you should start your journey toward recovery with intuitive eating and fitness. Only you can do that. I don't know what your particular story is, why you're reading this book, or how best to help you personally. Only you know that. I can only give to you the strategies I've learned from professionals in the field. I can only tell you my story and hope that parts of it resonate with you in a way that makes you feel less alone and hopeless. I do think recovery is possible for all people. As I said before, we only get one life, and we also don't know when it will end or what comes after. I would like to say we'll all die at an old age, but experience has taught me that such an end is a luxury, not a birthright.

So whatever you feel is right for you, do it with your whole heart, and do it with conviction. Do it with freedom.

---

41. Mike Morrison and Neal J. Roese, "Regrets of the Typical American: Findings from a Nationally Representative Sample," *Social Psychological and Personality Science* 2, no. 6 (March 2011): 576–583, https://doi.org/10.1177/1948550611401756.

Invitation to Join Me

To find out more about me and Freedom with Food and Fitness, visit www.freedomwithfoodandfitness.com, where I offer several virtual group-coaching packages to fit your needs, budget, and desired level of support.

There, you will also find my podcast, client testimonials, information on how to book me as a speaker, free intuitive-eating worksheets and videos, and information on how to work with me as your coach.

You can also connect with me on
Instagram @FreedomwithFoodandFitness.

Appendix: Recommended Reading List

Intuitive Eating by Evelyn Tribole and Elyse Resch

Health at Every Size: The Surprising Truth About Your Weight by Lindo Bacon

The Body Is Not an Apology: The Power of Radical Self-Love by Sonya Renee Taylor

Every Body Yoga: Let Go of Fear, Get on the Mat, Love Your Body by Jessamyn Stanley

Fearing the Black Body: The Racial Origins of Fat Phobia by Sabrina Strings, Allyson Johnson, et al.

The Beauty Myth by Naomi Wolf

Fat and Queer: An Anthology of Queer and Trans Bodies and Lives, edited by Bruce Owens Grimm, Miguel M. Morales, and Tiff Joshua TJ Ferentini

The F*ck It Diet by Caroline Dooner

Anti-Diet: Reclaim Your Time, Money, Well-Being, and Happiness Through Intuitive Eating by Christy Harrison

The Obesity Myth by Paul Campos

Shattered Image: My Triumph over Body Dysmorphic Disorder by Brian Cuban

Gender Outside the Binary: Eating Disorder Recovery and My Transgender Identity by Ryan K. Sallans, MA

Lesbian Crushes and Bulimia: A Diary on How I Acquired My Eating Disorder by Natasha Holme

Body Positive Power by Megan Jayne Crabbe

Works Cited

Arcelus, Jon, Alex J. Mitchell, Jackie Wales, et al. "Mortality Rates in Patients with Anorexia Nervosa and Other Eating Disorders: A Meta-analysis of 36 Studies." *Archives of General Psychiatry* 68, no. 7 (2011): 724–31.

Baker, David B., and Natacha Keramidas. "The Psychology of Hunger." *Monitor on Psychology* 44, no. 9 (October 2013): 66. http://www.apa.org/monitor/2013/10/hunger.

Becker, Anne E., Debra L. Franko, Alexandra Speck, and David B. Herzog. "Ethnicity and Differential Access to Care for Eating Disorder Symptoms." *International Journal of Eating Disorders* 33, no. 2 (March 2003): 205–12.

Brewerton, Timothy D. "Eating Disorders, Trauma, and Comorbidity: Focus on PTSD." *Eating Disorders* 15, no. 4 (August 2007): 285–304. https://doi.org/10.1080/10640260701454311.

Brown, Harriet. "The Obesity Paradox: Scientists Now Think That Being Overweight Can Protect Your Health." *Quartz*, November 17, 2015. http://qz.com/550527/obesity-paradox-scientists-now-think-that-being-overweight-is-sometimes-good-for-your-health/.

Caporuscio, Jessica. "What to Do About a Weight Loss Plateau." *Medical News Today*, September 23, 2019. https://www. medicalnewstoday.com/articles/326415.

Cherpak, Christine E. "Mindful Eating: A Review of How the Stress-Digestion-Mindfulness Triad May Modulate and Improve Gastrointestinal and Digestive Function." *Integrative Medicine* 18, no. 4 (August 2019): 48–53.

Curran, Thomas, and Andrew P. Hill. "Perfectionism Is Increasing over Time: A Meta-analysis of Birth Cohort Differences from 1989 to 2016." *Psychological Bulletin* 145, no. 4 (2019): 410–29. https://doi.org/10.1037/bul0000138.

Diener, Ed, and Martin E. P. Seligman. "Very Happy People." *Psychological Science* 13, no. 1 (January 2002): 81–84. https://doi.org/10.1111/1467-9280.00415.

Fernández-Elías, Valentín E., Juan F. Ortega, Rachael K. Nelson, and Ricardo Mora-Rodriguez. "Relationship between Muscle Water and Glycogen Recovery after Prolonged Exercise in the Heat in Humans." *European Journal of Applied Physiology* 115, no. 9 (September 2015): 1919–26. https://doi.org/10.1007/s00421-015-3175-z.

Flegal, Katherine M., Brian K. Kit, Heather Orpana, and Barry I. Graubard. "Association of All-Cause Mortality with Overweight and Obesity Using Standard Body Mass Index Categories: A Systematic Review and Meta-Analysis." *JAMA* 309, no. 1 (January 2013): 71–82. https://doi.org/10.1001/jama.2012.113905.

Fritsch, Jane. "95% Regain Lost Weight. Or Do They?" *New York Times*, May 25, 1999: F7. http://www.nytimes.com/1999/05/25/health/95-regain-lost-weight-or-do-they.html.

Gillen, Jenna B., Brian J. Martin, Martin J. MacInnis, Lauren E. Skelly, Mark A. Tarnopolsky, and Martin J. Gibala. "Twelve Weeks of Sprint Interval Training Improves Indices of Cardiometabolic Health Similar to Traditional Endurance Training Despite a Five-Fold Lower Exercise Volume and Time Commitment." *PLOS ONE* 11, no. 4 (April 2016): 1–14. https://doi.org/10.1371/journal.pone.0154075.

Gordon, Aubrey. "It's Time for a Culture of Consent Around Body Talk." *SELF*, August 27, 2020. http://www.self.com/story/body-talk-consent.

"How Common Is PTSD in Adults?" National Center for PTSD. U.S. Department of Veterans Affairs. Last modified April 8, 2022. http://www.ptsd.va.gov/understand/common/common_adults.asp.

Jung, Chang Hee, and Min-Seon Kim. "Molecular Mechanisms of Central Leptin Resistance in Obesity." *Archives of Pharmacal Research* 36, no. 2 (January 2013): 201–207. https://doi.org/10.1007/s12272-013-0020-y.

Lei, Xue, and David Perrett. "Misperceptions of Opposite-Sex Preferences for Thinness and Muscularity." *British Journal of Psychology* 112, no. 1 (May 2020): 247–61. https://doi.org/10.1111/bjop.12451.

Mann, Traci, A. Janet Tomiyama, Erika Westling, Ann-Marie Lew, Barbra Samuels, and Jason Chatman. "Medicare's Search for Effective Obesity Treatments: Diets Are Not the Answer." *American Psychologist* 62, no. 3 (April 2007): 220–33. https://doi.org/10.1037/0003-066X.62.3.220.

Matthews, Gail. "The Impact of Commitment, Accountability, and Written Goals on Goal Achievement." Dominican University

Psychology Faculty Presentation, 2007. https://scholar.
dominican.edu/psychology-faculty-conference-presentations/3/.

McCabe, David P., and Alan D. Castel. "Seeing Is Believing: The
Effect of Brain Images on Judgments of Scientific Reasoning."
Cognition 107, no. 1 (April 2008): 343–52. https://doi.
org/10.1016/j.cognition.2007.07.017.

McCarthy, Mandy. "The Thin Ideal, Depression and Eating
Disorders in Women." *Behaviour Research and Therapy* 28, no.
3 (1990): 205–14. https://doi.
org/10.1016/0005-7967(90)90003-2.

Moran, Alyssa J., Maricelle Ramirez, and Jason P. Block. "Consumer
Underestimation of Sodium in Fast Food Restaurant Meals:
Results from a Cross-Sectional Observational Study." *Appetite*
113 (June 2017): 155–61. https://doi.org/10.1016/j.
appet.2017.02.028.

Morrison, Mike, and Neal J. Roese. "Regrets of the Typical
American: Findings from a Nationally Representative Sample."
Social Psychological and Personality Science 2, no. 6 (March
2011): 576–583. https://doi.org/10.1177/1948550611401756.

Müller, Manfred J., Anya Bosy-Westphal, and Steven B. Heymsfield.
"Is There Evidence for a Set Point that Regulates Human Body
Weight?" *F1000 Medicine Reports* 2, no. 59 (August 2010): 1-7.
https://doi.org/10.3410/M2-59.

Pedram, Pardis, Danny Wadden, Peyvand Amini, Wayne Gulliver,
Edward Randell, et al. "Food Addiction: Its Prevalence and
Significant Association with Obesity in the General Population."
PLOS ONE 8, no. 9 (September 2013): 1–6. https://doi.
org/10.1371/journal.pone.0074832.

Phillips, Katharine A. "Body Dysmorphic Disorder: Recognizing and Treating Imagined Ugliness." *World Psychiatry* 3, no. 1 (February 2004): 12–17.

Reichelt, Amy. "Your Brain on Sugar: What the Science Actually Says." *The Conversation*, November 14, 2019. https:// theconversation.com/ your-brain-on-sugar-what-the-science-actually says-126581.

Romero-Corral, Abel, Virend K. Somers, Justo Sierra-Johnson, Randal J. Thomas, Kent R. Bailey, Maria L. Collazo-Clavell, Thomas G. Allison, Josef Korinek, John A. Batsis, F. H. Sert-Kuniyoshi, and Francisco Lopez-Jimenez. "Accuracy of Body Mass Index in Diagnosing Obesity in the Adult General Population." *International Journal of Obesity* 32, no. 6 (July 2008): 959–66. https://doi.org/10.1038/ijo.2008.11.

Ross, Robert, Bret H. Goodpaster, Lauren G. Koch, Mark A. Sarzynski, Wendy M. Kohrt, Neil M. Johannsen, James S. Skinner, et al. "Precision Exercise Medicine: Understanding Exercise Response Variability." *British Journal of Sports Medicine* 53, no. 18 (March 2019): 1141–53. http://dx.doi. org/10.1136/bjsports-2018-100328.

Rustagi, Neeti, S. K. Pradhan, and Ritesh Singh, "Public Health Impact of Plastics: An Overview." *Indian Journal of Occupational and Environmental Medicine* 15, no. 3 (2011): 100–103. https://doi.org/10.4103/0019-5278.93198.

Schimel, Jeff, Jamie Arndt, Tom Pyszczynski, and Jeff Greenberg. "Being Accepted for Who We Are: Evidence that Social Validation of the Intrinsic Self Reduces General Defensiveness." *Journal of Personality and Social Psychology*

80, no. 1 (January 2001): 35–52. https://doi.
org/10.1037//0022-3514.80.1.35.

Selig, Meg. "Why Diets Don't Work … and What Does." *Psychology Today*, October 21, 2010. http://www.psychologytoday.com/us/
blog/changepower/201010/why-diets-dont-work-and-what-does.

Sencer. "Is Milk Good or Bad for You?" *KQED*, March 9, 2016.
http://www.kqed.org/education/130193/
is-milk-good-or-bad-for-you.

Soares, Fabíola Lacerda Pires, Mariana Herzog Ramos, Mariana
Gramelisch, Rhaviny de Paula Pego Silva, Jussara da Silva
Batista, Monica Cattafesta, and Luciane Bresciani Salaroli.
"Intuitive Eating Is Associated with Glycemic Control in Type
2 Diabetes." *Eating and Weight Disorders* 26, no. 2 (March
2021): 599–608. https://doi.org/10.1007/
s40519-020-00894-8.

Stamp, Rebecca. "Average Person Will Try 126 Fad Diets in Their
Lifetime, Poll Claims." *Independent*, January 8, 2020. https://
www.independent.co.uk/life-style/diet-weight-loss-food-
unhealthy-eating-habits-a9274676.html.

Stunkard, Albert, and Mavis McLaren-Hume. "The Results of
Treatment for Obesity: A Review of the Literature and Report of
a Series." *AMA Archives of Internal Medicine* 103, no. 1
(January 1959): 79–85. https://doi.org/10.1001/
archinte.1959.00270010085011.

Swart, Tara, Kitty Chisholm, and Paul Brown. *Neuroscience for
Leadership: Harnessing the Brain Gain Advantage*. New York:
Palgrave Macmillan, 2015.

"U.S. Weight Loss & Diet Control Market Report 2021: Market
    Reached a Record $78 Billion in 2019, but Suffered a 21%
    Decline in 2020 Due to COVID-19 – Forecast to 2025 –
    ResearchAndMarkets.com." *Business Wire*, March 26, 2021.
    https://www.businesswire.com/news/home/20210326005126/
    en/U.S.-Weight-Loss-Diet-Control-Market-Report-2021-Market-
    Reached-a-Record-78-Billion-in-2019-but-Suffered-a-21-Decline-
    in-2020-Due-to-COVID-19---Forecast-to-2025---
    ResearchAndMarkets.com.

Wheless, James W. "History of the Ketogenic Diet." *Epilepsia* 49,
    suppl. 8 (November 2008): 3–5. https://doi.
    org/10.1111/j.1528-1167.2008.01821.x.

"Why People Become Overweight." *Harvard Health Publishing*,
    June 24, 2019. https://www.health.harvard.edu/staying-healthy/
    why-people-become-overweight.